April 10, 1990

To- Joanne
        With love,
            Mother

" I asked the birds
To sing for you
I asked the sun
To smile on you
I asked God to send
His love to you
On this your "Special"
        day!

Nourishing the Life Force

By Richard and Mary-Alice Jafolla

Unity Books
Unity Village, Missouri

Cover photograph by
Norman Poole
Gastonia, NC

Third Printing 1985

Contents

Introduction

Dear Friend,

God expresses in the body temple as the life force which knows and seeks only health and wholeness. The thoughts we think and the foods we eat nourish that life force and affect the chemistry of the body temple. We have an unlimited potential for expression, but we can never be more than what we believe ourselves to be. Nor can our bodies ever build tissues better than the raw materials we have given them to build with! The dynamics of the mind must work with the chemistry of the body if we are to allow the life force to bring forth perfect health.

This book is meant to serve as one means of working with the life force. You can use it in either of two ways. It can be read in total as a treatise on healing and health. Or it can be used as a reference book to offer aid for a specific challenge you may now be facing. In whatever manner you choose to use the book, we urge you to pay special attention to the first, second, and last chapters.

If you have been searching for the answers to your health challenge, perhaps the ideas set forth in this book may help to launch your rebirth.

The Authors

The Body Temple

Charles Fillmore once wrote: *The real body of God is a living body. Above all, it is a beautiful body, a temple. And God Himself is in that temple. . . .*

The marvels, the intricacies, and the splendor of just one tiny cell of this temple would put to shame 10,000 temples of Solomon, so awesome are the structure and function of our body temples, so *fearfully and wonderfully made* are we.

What man-made edifice could ever match the inscrutable network of human tissues arranged so perfectly by Divine Mind seeking to live through us—through us and as us?

Oh, the miracle of it all—this human body, the most magnificent manifestation of all creation, that begins with an individual cell and develops by divine design into an individual being! The more one learns of the mysteries lying deep within our cellular membranes, the more one bows in humble worship to the almighty Creator who so obviously dwells within those membranes.

Pause for a few moments right now and think of all the wonders that go on in the body—routinely and without our conscious direction.

Dear friends, we are such works as no human hands could ever fashion nor human mind ever envision. We are the work and dwelling-place of God, each of us a holy temple filled with Spirit seeking perfection and life. And once entrusted with the sacred gift of life, each of us must do his part to maintain that life and keep his temple befitting of the majesty that resides there.

Man's body temple is the outer expression of the Garden of Eden, which God gave him to keep and to trim. This too from Charles Fillmore, a man in many ways ahead of his time in recognizing the need for constant care of the physical body temple.

Today more than ever before we are discovering the Truth about the body temple and how specific laws decreed by the Creator must be obeyed if we are to attain that state of perfect health for which the temple was created.

The fact that we may not have reached a state of perfect health should not discourage us. The important thing to realize is that perfect health is attainable. It is attainable because there is, flowing through us, a universal life force, and this force is always seeking perfection.

Have you ever wondered why a broken bone mends; why a cut tissue heals; why a pulled muscle is repaired; why, when we sense danger, we are nudged to change our plans toward a more prudent path? Why? Because there is a special force that wants us to be perfect and will not be satisfied until we are perfect.

This is the force with which the healing arts work. A physician does not "cure" you of a sickness. He merely uses skillful, time-tested techniques that temporarily slow down the malady—delay it—until the body can rally its own resources. For the true cure comes from within the body itself, not from something done to the body from without.

Sickness Is Not Natural

Lack of health is not prevalent in God's universe. If such lack appears anywhere it is the work of man. Charles Fillmore has identified the problem most succinctly. Because a lack of health is "apparent" does not mean it is "normal." If there is a lack of health in our lives, let us not look toward the outer to ascertain its cause; let us look within at the "work of man" and see what we have done to cause it.

Our bodies are self-regulating, self-repairing, self-renewing organisms that have only one passionate, all-encompassing, overriding desire—and that is *to live!* Our bodies know nothing of sickness, nothing of disease, nothing of death. Our bodies know only life and seek only life. To subject them to thoughts of disease and death is to pervert them. It is to deny the existence of the universal life force that flows through us, ever seeking and ever guiding our bodies toward perfection.

Spirit, soul, and body are the three phases of humanity. This idea is among the oldest doctrines of philosophy. There is a balance which is necessary—which is crucial—among these three phases. There has been a tendency, especially among some New Thought students, to minimize the importance of the body—an inclination to ignore the body and to concentrate instead on improving the mind. This is dangerous, for a balance is needed. Charles Fillmore tells us: *To give men opportunity to get the full benefit of salvation, life is necessary, and a body through which to express life is also necessary.* In His ministry Jesus did not ignore the flesh. When Jesus healed, His healings were of mind and body jointly.

Myrtle Fillmore once wrote: *Evidently, the individual soul has felt the need of just such an earth home as the body temple. We are to realize that the body, free from the inharmonies and weaknesses imposed upon it through error, is a part of God's plan of life.*

How can we express our divinity without a body? When we lose our body, we also lose our brain and nervous system. Charles Fillmore warns us: *When a man relin-*

3

*quishes his hold on brain and nervous system, he gives up
the only avenue through which he can adequately express
himself.*

Yes, the body is as important as the other phases of
our being. There is a perfect relationship among all three in
Divine Mind, and that is what we should strive to attain.

Temple of God

The fact that God dwells within us makes our bodies
holy temples. Within the body's inner precincts, within
every organ, every tissue, within every cell, dwells its
Creator.

The Old Testament put a great deal of stress on the
temple. Metaphysically, the temple represents the body.
The first temple in the Bible was a tent. This was the best
that the Children of Israel could do at that time. However,
years later when Solomon became king, history tells us he
built a Temple of such magnificence and splendor that it has
never been equaled.

Unfortunately, some people still have a "tent" consciousness when it comes to their bodies. They are satisfied
with the most minimum structure—a structure that is constantly being torn and tattered by the vicissitudes of life and
has little chance of any permanence.

How much more meaningful it is to present our
Creator with a structure that, when properly cared for,
makes Solomon's Temple pale in comparison. Such is the
human body—the supreme treasure of creation, the rarest
of jewels.

In one of her many letters, Myrtle Fillmore wrote:
*Sometimes we fail to remember that the temple is for the
use of the Holy Spirit.* This is something we must always
remember. Within us dwells our Creator!

It is our responsibility to make our bodies fit dwelling places for God. It is our responsibility to maintain and repair our temples, and we can do this only by obeying those laws of body maintenance that an all-wise Creator has established. For there are definite laws that govern the care of the body, and it is incumbent on each individual to ascertain these laws and to conscientiously employ them.

No one would deny that there is great order in the universe. This order is maintained by very definite laws. The same laws that apply to the orbits of the stars and planets in deepest space apply just as fully to the electrons and protons in the atoms deep within our bodies. It must be so. What kind of chaos would prevail if a Creator changed laws to suit every cry of discontent from one of His creations? The universe must have rules, must have laws, if it is to survive. And, if we are to survive, we must learn and obey these laws.

Science has discovered a great many universal laws. We usually refer to these as "physical laws." However, let us not fall into the mistaken belief that these physical laws are somehow inferior to spiritual or mental laws. There is no hierarchy of laws in the universe. There is no one law in nature that contradicts another. Nature is not in conflict with itself.

In reality there are no "physical" laws and "mental" laws and "spiritual" laws—there are only *God's* laws. Every new discovery in physics or chemistry or medicine is as much a revelation of God's laws as is the most sublime theological insight.

If we obey God's laws, we fit perfectly into the divine mosaic of universal perfection, and we experience perfection in all phases of life. If we attempt to violate these laws, we suffer to the exact extent of our indiscretion. Charles Fillmore put it best when he said: *The sin, sickness, suffer-*

ing, and death that men experience are not punishment willed by God; they are results of broken law. The law is good; men have joy, satisfaction, and life in everlasting harmony when they keep the law. Creation would not be possible without rules governing the created.*

Body Chemistry

The body is governed by the same laws that govern chemistry. The body is, in fact, a chemical compound. We are a swarming sea of chemical reactions—billions every second—and the atoms involved in these reactions follow the same rules, the same laws, as every other atom in the universe. The protein that gives your tissues the unique shape that is you is made up of the same carbon, hydrogen, oxygen, and nitrogen that are part of the farthest star. The trace amount of iodine in your thyroid gland is exactly the same as the iodine found in the ocean depths. The iron in your blood, which delivers oxygen to your waiting cells, is the same iron that can be found in the very bowels of the Earth. The laws of chemistry governing the human body are as inviolable as those governing the rest of the universe.

The thoughts we think and the foods we eat affect our body chemistry. Discordant thoughts yield discordant body chemistry; discordant food yields discordant body chemistry; and discordant body chemistry yields "sickness." It is as elementary as that! We are dealing with the law of cause and effect.

Charles and Myrtle Fillmore were aware of the importance of both food and thought. On one occasion Charles said: . . . *we should spiritualize our thoughts and refine the food we eat to correspond.* Myrtle wrote: *We must know the chemistry of the body. We must feed the whole man. . . . Learn what it* [the body] *needs and arrange for supplying those needs.*

In trying to determine what the body needs, it is crucial to realize that we are a society of cells. Each of us is composed of about 100 trillion little "beings," each imbued with a divine intelligence and each seeking wholeness, health, and perfection.

Life begins at the cellular level. Each of the lifeless elements that we take into the body in the form of food and drink remains lifeless until it is incorporated into the cells. Once within their inner sanctum, the cells, following a divine blueprint, perform the miraculous chemical wizardry necessary to distill these inert elements into the supreme treasure of the universe—life!

Within each cell there is a divine plan for perfection—there is an intelligence. Our cells want wholeness; they want health; our cells want life.

Every cell of the body is enveloped in soul or thought, and its initial impulse is to conform to the divine-natural law. This, from Charles Fillmore. Unless we become aware of our cellular needs, we run the risk of working at cross-purposes with them.

If we are interested in life and health, then we must learn to work in concert with this cellular intelligence. It is the only way.

Health—an Inside Job

Probably the most important thing we can do to change our health is to realize that it is *we* who decide just what our health will be. If we want to be healthy, if health is our *true* desire, then the first thing we have to do is to let our mental and spiritual attitudes mirror that desire. This should be our primary consideration. All else follows the desire for health. And it must follow closely, for a desire

7

without a deed is a dead end.

And what kinds of deeds are needed? When our mental outlook is adjusted to think in terms of health and life, our attention must then turn to our physical actions, especially eating and exercise.

Exercise

It is not within the purview of this book to deal extensively with exercise. However, it is good to keep in mind that no matter how highly nutritious the foods we eat, if the nutrients from them fail to reach the cells then we are, in fact, poorly nourished! The only way for any nutrients to reach our cells is by circulation through the blood and lymphatic system. And it is a fact that exercise is the best way to improve circulation. Without exercise, the entire system—not only the circulatory system—will slow down and stagnate. Nutrients will not be delivered to waiting cells, and poor health will ensue.

In addition to helping to distribute nutrients, exercise has many other values, not the least of which is its effect on the nervous system. Exercise can bring about a significant tranquilizing effect as proficiently as any drug, but without the dangerous side effects. (Indeed, the side effects of exercise are a stronger heart, greater lung capacity, and better neuromuscular function!) And the exercise need not be strenuous to be effective.

There are many forms of exercise available, and most people know which ones are best for them. Almost all forms of mild exercises are beneficial, especially rhythmic exercises. Walking is especially good. After only one month of regular, brisk, daily walks in the fresh air, you will see and feel a delicious difference in your body and in your mind. You will look better, feel better, think better, and sleep better. Your brain will be more alert and you will have more energy to meet each day.

Choose an exercise and *do it regularly*. Regularity is the key. An exercise that can be done in the fresh air is better than one that must be done indoors. Remember, an exercise does not have to be strenuous to be beneficial. Some other good exercises, in addition to walking are: jogging, rope skipping, swimming, bicycling, rowing, square dancing, yoga, tennis, golfing, and many, many others. The exercise you choose should raise your heart rate about fifty percent and sustain that rate for at least twenty to thirty minutes each time you exercise. And you should try to exercise every day. If this is not possible, do it at least four days each week. (Of course, it is always best to check with your physician before beginning any exercise program.)

Keep in mind that muscles were designed to move and to move regularly. In fact, you must move them if you are to improve them. A good exercise program is a solid investment in your future, one that will pay rich dividends.

Nutrition

The great Roman statesman Seneca said: *We dig our graves with our teeth*. Two thousand years ago people knew that food was intimately related to health. Judging from the advertisements on TV and a walk along the aisles of a supermarket, we seem to have forgotten this simple fact. *The food we eat affects the chemistry of our bodies.* If we choose to put wholesome foods into our bodies, then they will respond with health and vigor. If we put harmful foods into our bodies, they will respond in sickness and lassitude. The choice is ours.

It may seem to contradict the laws of mind to say that we can do nothing to ameliorate the consequences of poor

9

eating habits. Why can't we just eat what we want to eat, deny that there is anything in the food that will harm us, and then affirm health for our bodies? Surely if we deny with enough vehemence and affirm with enough faith, we can change the bad effects of the food?

But how can we really believe this? Isn't that a contradiction of the law of compensation? How can we believe that the law of compensation applies to every atom in the universe but not to us? Richard Lynch put it well when he wrote: *To believe blindly that some mysterious power outside the body is going to descend upon and vitalize it . . . [after we have disobeyed God's] orderly laws, is not only futile but unintelligent.* We just cannot attempt to break physical laws and get away with it.

But then the question arises, "How did Jesus perform His miracles if He was not breaking physical laws?" Jesus did not break physical laws any more than we break the law of gravity when we fly. The law of gravity is very much in effect when we're airborne; however, the airplane is responding to the laws of aerodynamics. These are not *higher* laws than the law of gravity, they are merely *other* laws. Both are equally valid. We can choose which we want to use at the appropriate time. When a pilot wants to ascend, he utilizes the laws of aerodynamics. When he wants to descend, he utilizes the laws of gravity.

Jesus performed feats that seem to contradict the physical laws as we know them. But they were not really contradictory. In walking on water, raising the dead, healing the blind, and even in resurrecting His own body, Jesus was not using "higher" laws than physical laws. But it is important to remember that Jesus had a consciousness that differed from ours—that is the crucial key. And it is different from ours because He had a consciousness that did not rely on His senses but rather on His Spirit. He did not believe that because He could "feel" someone's withered arm He could not fill it out. He did not believe that because He could "hear" that leprosy was incurable He could not heal it. He did not believe that because He could "see" that Lazarus was dead He could not raise him. His consciousness was not bounded by His senses. He had a consciousness that expanded to the very boundaries of His Spirit and was, therefore, limitless. And acting within that limitless consciousness He did not accept any condition as "terminal." To the consciousness of Jesus, as witnessed by Lazarus, Jairus's daughter, and others, not even death itself was a terminal condition!

But we have limited our consciousness. By adopting attitudes such as "seeing is believing," we set outer limits for our consciousness and so restrict it that we can only function within its boundaries. Jesus had a consciousness that was not bounded and so He could act as one with the universe. On the other hand, because we have limited ourselves by our false beliefs, *we can only function within the self-imposed boundaries of our present consciousness.* So if, *in your present consciousness,* you need an airplane to fly, then don't try to get out of the airplane ten minutes before it lands, no matter how much you have denied the effects of the law of gravity. If, *in your present consciousness,* you need a boat under you to stay above the water, don't try to walk on the water, no matter how much you deny the laws of hydrostatics. If, *in your present consciousness,* you must eat food in order to live, don't eat harmful food and expect to be healthy, no matter how strongly you deny the laws of nutrition. *We can only function within the self-imposed boundaries of our present consciousness.*

The authors are assuming that everyone reading this book must ingest food and drink in order to live. If this is so, then you must obey the laws of nutrition if you are to be well. Now, this is not to say that eating, by itself, will engender health. As we mentioned earlier, the primary task is to change your mental and spiritual outlook. When you do this, all else follows. Read what Charles Fillmore had to say about this: . . . *when we ask and by affirmation proclaim its presence,* [the Spirit of truth] *brings new life into our body and moves us to observe hygienic and dietary laws that restore health.*

Tithe Your Food

Those who know the dynamics of giving and receiving are aware of the fact that as one freely and lovingly gives, one can expect a manifold return on that gift. This is the dynamics of tithing. We give a portion of our good, knowing that it and more will be returned to us.

We can and should use the same concept in dealing with the food we eat. As we choose good, wholesome food to rebuild our precious cells, we should claim a return of health from it. And why not? As we ingest these rich and natural foods, they disperse their nutrients deep within the body to nurture us and keep us well. Charles Fillmore wrote: *No one has ever seen life in food or drink, but it is there in small degree, and it is through eating and drinking that the body absorbs the invisible life elements. . . . Anytime we eat good food, we are making an investment in our health.*

Choose well from the foods God has provided. Bless the wonderful food as you eat it, and claim your rightful return of health from it. A word of caution, however: You can claim your good only from wholesome food. To try to claim a return of health from unwholesome food would be like putting a bad check in the collection plate on Sunday and trying to claim a tenfold return of prosperity!

Like the prodigal son who returned home to claim his birthright—abundant riches—our bodies want to return to their true home and claim their divine birthright—abundant health. And we can help by cooperating with the divine intelligence within each cell. Remember, however, that when we speak of rights, we must speak of responsibilities. If we forfeit our responsibility to health, we forfeit our rights to it.

In forthcoming chapters we will be specific as to what we all can do to work with our life force. We will list the five nutritional essentials to health, and we will offer specific suggestions on problems such as overweight, depression, arthritis, low blood sugar, diabetes, and many more.

In the meantime, you can begin today to communicate with your cells. The first thing to do is what you would do to anyone whom you've abused—apologize. Apologize for all the past nutritional "sins" you have committed against your cells. Know that these nutritional indiscretions are now behind you and that you won't commit them again. From this day onward you will treat the precious cells in your body like the diminutive divinities they are.

It is never too late to begin the quest for perfect health. After all, our cells are constantly renewing themselves. We are miracle machines whose parts rebuild and renew. We don't get older—we get newer! The finer the material we put into the body, the finer the quality of that body.

Make a commitment to good health. Be aware that as long as you honor your commitment, good health will ensue.

An excellent way to make a true commitment is to establish a covenant. You can make a sacred covenant with your life force and promise to do your share, knowing that if you do, the life force will certainly do its share.

A "Covenant with the Life Force" has been included here for you to use if you wish.

Covenant with the Life Force

Father-Mother God, Creator of the universe, Lord of my being, I acknowledge Your power as the source of my life, Your intelligence as the director of my cells, Your substance as the fiber of my tissues. I give thanks for Your life force within me, and I apologize for my past mistreatment of Your holy temple — my body. I know now that I must work with Your life force if I am to fully express my potential for perfection.

Therefore, on this _____ day of _____, 19____, I do earnestly and joyfully make this covenant with the life force manifesting in my cells:

I promise to appropriate into my mind only thoughts of health and wholeness, envisioning my cells as the perfection they were created to be — worthy of my most noble attitudes and aspirations.

I promise to appropriate into my body only foods of health and wholeness, knowing that God resides in the foods He created, and knowing, too, that what I eat today I become tomorrow.

I promise to appropriate into my life-style only actions of health and wholeness. To this extent I will seek abundant fresh air and adequate rest; and I will engage in regular constructive exercises, knowing that as I move a muscle, I improve that muscle, and that what is constantly improved cannot perish.

I enter into this covenant in the full realization that God's laws are inviolable. I have unshakable faith in the fact that as long as I honor my commitments to perfection, the universe will follow inexorably its law of cause and effect and will reward me with the unlimited health and wholeness I so fervently seek and desire.

_____
Signature

Your Body's Nutritional Needs

In the preceding chapter, we said that wholeness and health are our natural state. However, we also pointed out that it is incumbent on us to obey the laws that an all-wise Creator has formulated to keep order in the universe if we expect to possess health and wholeness.

We determined that the physical laws were as inviolable as any other laws, and that ultimately all laws are God's laws and must be followed.

The body was depicted as a society of cells, each having an intelligence and each possessing a divine blueprint for life and health. It is to these cells that we must address our nutritional needs.

The 100 trillion cells that make us up follow the laws of chemistry. The foods we eat and the thoughts we think affect body chemistry. We decide our state of health by choosing which thoughts and nutrients we appropriate into our bodies. Denials and affirmations alone are not enough, nor is desire alone. A desire without a deed is a dead end.

One of the key points mentioned was that we must function within the boundaries of our present consciousness. If in our present consciousness we must have food and drink in order to live, then we had better be sure that we choose the finest foods and the finest beverages. Existing on the physical plane means obeying physical laws.

The universe has provided us with a plethora of foods from which to choose. One would think that with the thousands of foods available to us we would be content to choose from these. But, alas, it just is not so. Not content with the one mistake we made in the allegory about the apple in the Garden of Eden, we compound that mistake by taking the wonderful apple and making apple pie! Not content with cow's milk, we make ice cream. Not content with grains, we make whiskey. Are these the foods that God has presented to us to nurture His most wonderful creation? Do you really believe that the miracle machine that is your body was designed to function on such counterfeit foods as coffee, pastries, soft drinks, sugar, white flour, cookies, cakes, and the like? We are responsible for the perversions of the food God made!

We are fortunate to live in an age when science has given us a list of essential nutrients—things the body needs to repair and renew itself. We mustn't make the mistake of demeaning scientific discoveries; they are as much a revelation of God's laws as are the most incisive eschatological and theological insights. Myrtle Fillmore wrote: . . . *we need to make practical all the knowledge we have concerning bodily renewal, through using intelligence and discrimination in the selection of our food.*

Science tells us that for an optimum diet we need, every day, adequate amounts of the following: protein, carbohydrates, oils, minerals, and vitamins. (There are actually six nutritional essentials if we include water. We assume, however, that most everyone gets enough of this critical nutrient and, therefore, we will not include it for discussion.) If we get these nutrients in optimum amounts every day, we have satisfied our nutritional requirements. (Of course, we still need regular exercise, adequate rest, fresh air, and sunshine.)

Looks simple, doesn't it? Well, it is simple, although it may not be easy. And it may not be easy because we have allowed our food selection to be dominated by the relatively few primitive cells that make up our taste buds. We are too

16

interested in what it *tastes* like instead of what it will do for us, so we allow the taste buds to dictate our eating habits. But it is a serious mistake to choose our food on the basis of its entertainment value alone. We must not live under the tyranny of the taste buds. We have been given an intellect with which to make decisions. When we allow a few cells to usurp the decision-making capabilities of the brain, we borrow trouble for the body. The food we appropriate into our bodies is every bit as important as the thoughts we appropriate into our minds. What we *think* today, we become tomorrow. What we *eat* today, we become tomorrow. Let us choose our thoughts and our foods with the utmost care.

(Editor's note: You may wish to leave a marker at the beginning of the next section, as you will be advised to refer to it often throughout the book.)

Protein — The First Essential

The importance of protein is indicated by the fact that it comes from the Greek *proteios* meaning "primary" or "of first importance." The importance of protein—the proper kinds and in the proper amounts—cannot be overemphasized. No body can sustain itself, much less rebuild itself, without the ingestion of protein. Next to water it is the most abundant substance in the body.

One look in the mirror will tell us why. All that we see is protein tissue—skin, hair, eyes, ears. If we smile, we'll see more protein tissue—gums, tongue, and even tooth enamel contain some!

But protein does not stop at the exterior of the body. The brain contains protein, as do the lungs, the heart, the nerves, the glands, and the disks between our vertebrae. Our male and female hormones and the hormone insulin are also composed of protein as is about ninety-five percent

17

of the hemoglobin molecule.

Put very simply, life requires protein! It is an indispensable and normal constituent of every living cell. God builds tissue with the bricks and mortar of protein. Without protein there can be no repairing, rebuilding, or renewing.

We can't really understand protein properly unless we understand amino acids, the chemical units out of which proteins are made. These are the building blocks, or the divine alphabet, of protein which the Creator uses to construct life. There are about twenty-two in all that concern us. Just as we can make millions of words out of our twenty-six letter alphabet, so can there be an almost infinite number of proteins made from the amino acids.

Of the twenty-two amino acids, the adult human body can make all but eight. These eight are called the *essential amino acids;* and, since we cannot make them, they must be obtained in the foods we eat. Foods containing all eight of these essential amino acids are called *complete proteins.* If it is lacking or in short supply of even one of these eight, it is an *incomplete protein.* We of course will choose only from the complete proteins. (Incomplete proteins can be eaten, certainly; but we will not count them in our daily protein total.)

The list of primary or top-grade proteins is rather short. The top-grade proteins are the ones that are not only "complete" but that have the best balance of amino acids.

The finest protein and the one to which the biochemists have assigned the highest biological activity is that humble single cell of potential life—the egg. The egg is the finest protein food available. Next comes milk, another great protein. (Included with milk are skimmed milk, goat milk, yogurt, kefir, and others.)

Slightly lower than milk but still a top-grade protein is the protein in cheese. This includes all of the hard cheeses

(Swiss, cheddar, jack) and many of the soft cheeses (such as farmers, mozzarella, and cottage cheese).

Last on the list are lean meat, fish, and poultry. These do not have the high biological activity of the others but still must be considered top-grade proteins.

Now, in considering this list, be sure to realize that you do not have to eat all these proteins in order to be healthy. Vegetarians would not be interested in the last group, and that is fine. They must then choose from the others. Some don't like to eat eggs; others don't like milk; and that is fine also. The important thing is to choose your proteins from this list. Choose one, or two, or all of them. These are the foods into which God has put His finest building materials. These are the foods with which we can most readily rebuild and renew the body. And remember, what is constantly renewed cannot perish.

How Much Is Enough?

In order to assure a proper daily intake of protein, we should strive to ingest about one gram of top-grade protein for *every two pounds* of *ideal* body weight. Thus, if our ideal weight is 120 pounds, we should try to get about sixty grams per day. If our ideal weight is 150 pounds, then we should try to ingest about seventy-five grams per day.

In order to count properly, this little chart should be memorized:

1 egg = 6 grams of protein
1 oz. of milk (including yogurt, kefir, goat milk) = 1 gram
1 oz. cheese = 7 grams (cottage cheese = about 4 grams)
1 oz. meat, fish, or poultry = 5 grams

These figures are, of course, approximations.

Use this chart every day. Be sure you are getting enough protein in your diet and counting in your daily totals only the top-grade proteins listed. Whole grains, nuts, seeds, and many other protein sources are wonderful foods and may be eaten regularly; but, unless they are combined intelligently, the protein content is inferior to the top-grade proteins and should not be counted in your daily total.

Remember, protein is the nutritional key to health. As we have already mentioned, God builds with the bricks and mortar of protein. The finer the quality of the bricks and mortar, the more magnificent will the temple become.

Constructive Carbohydrates

The word *constructive* is important when dealing with carbohydrates because eating the nonconstructive carbohydrates is the primary nutritional reason people get into physical trouble. Those carbohydrates that are not constructive are destructive. They work at cross-purposes to our indwelling life force. Instead of building health they will quickly destroy it.

Carbohydrates provide fuel for the body and an adequate supply is crucial to the proper functioning of the brain and nervous system, . . . *the only avenue through which* [man] *can adequately express himself,* said Charles Fillmore.

In addition to supplying us with energy, some carbohydrates determine what kinds of bacteria will grow in our intestines (friendly or unfriendly). Some will allow us to use fat more efficiently, while other carbohydrates will help us maintain normal bowel movements.

Carbohydrates also have a "protein-sparing action." We know the importance of protein's role in renewing our tissues. If the body does not have enough carbohydrates, it will be forced to use the protein for fuel, since it puts its need for energy above every other need—even the need to rebuild! When the protein is used for fuel, it cannot be used for rebuilding and renewing.

When sufficient amounts of carbohydrates are present in the diet, however, the body will utilize these carbohydrates as fuel and will allow the protein to go about its important task of renewing us.

Keep in mind that when we say "carbohydrates" we are referring to *constructive* carbohydrates. Carbohydrates are the food group where we can make our biggest nutritional errors. We tend to consume too many *destructive* carbohydrates. Our society seems geared to counterfeit foods: sugar, white flour, candy, cakes, pastry, soft drinks, alcohol, artificial sweeteners, diet drinks, and others. These are not body builders.

And what are the legitimate carbohydrates? The actual list of constructive carbohydrates (note the word "constructive") seems very short. In reality it is not. The list of constructive carbohydrates is:

Fresh fruit (apples, bananas, melons, peaches, etc.)
Fresh vegetables (squashes, peas, salad greens,
      potatoes, etc.)
Whole grains (wheat, rye, barley, rice, whole grain
      bread, etc.)
Honey, blackstrap molasses, and maple syrup (pure).

The last three on the list are very concentrated in natural sugar and should be used sparingly, if at all. The finest carbohydrates are the first three: fresh fruits, fresh vegetables, and whole grains. These are the carbohydrates bursting with life. These are the carbohydrates that the life force dwelling within us can work with to strengthen us and make us whole and healthy.

Fruits, vegetables, and grains are truly "health foods." Apples, pears, peaches, pineapples, melons, papayas, bananas, and all the other wonderful fruits are joyously welcomed by cells eager for such superb raw materials. The green peas, squashes, tomatoes, salad greens, carrots, string beans, potatoes, and all the other nourishing fresh vegetables are hungrily grabbed by cells intent on health and wholeness. The whole grains (including whole grain breads), such as wheat, rye, millet, rice, barley, oats, and many others are enthusiastically utilized by cells eager for life.

And as a bonus, fruits, vegetables, and grains are also wonderful for the health of the colon. Because the cellulose contained in all three is mostly indigestible, it acts as an excellent bulk. This bulk stimulates the lining of the intestines and induces peristalsis—the rhythmical contraction of the intestines which propels the intestinal contents onward and outward. Without the proper amount of bulk these foods give to the body, peristalsis will not occur and the toxins will not be forced out of the colon.

Just as we must use the technique of "denials" to rid ourselves of the toxic wastes of the past in order to make room for "affirming" good for our future, so the body must rid itself of the toxic wastes of its past metabolism to make room for more of the life-giving nutrients in its future.

Choose a carbohydrate for each meal; but choose carefully, for your body wants and deserves only the finest.

Oils for the Miracle Machine

No meal is complete merely with protein and carbohydrates. There is yet another essential food that the cells are waiting for, and that is fatty-acids, better known as oils. Each meal should include a good source of oil. The oil can be in the form of a good, unhydrogenated vegetable oil, or it can be a marvelously nutritious but not so fine-tasting oil like cod liver oil or wheat germ oil. (Luckily, these two are available in capsule form so our taste buds won't think they are being punished!)

Fats, especially the polyunsaturated oils, are essential to the body for many reasons. They are necessary for a multitude of metabolic functions including growth and reproduction, utilization of the fat-soluble vitamins (A, D, E, and K), and as a source of sustained energy.

If you are puzzled as to a pleasant way to get oil into every meal, find a good-tasting vegetable oil and use it for your salad dressing. It is also good on baked potatoes, in soups, and on cooked vegetables. Try some on your whole grain toast in the morning. It tastes like melted butter and is so much better for you.

Some excellent vegetable oils are: safflower oil, sunflower oil, English walnut oil, corn oil, and sesame oil. Find one you like and use it regularly.

If you still find it difficult to obtain enough good oil, you can supplement your diet with cod liver oil or wheat germ oil capsules.

One caveat about oils is worth mentioning. It is very easy to buy an inferior oil. Good oils are very fragile and, in nature, are protected by natural antioxidants, such as vitamin E. However, when they are extracted from the safflower or corn or whatever, the natural antioxidants are destroyed or removed. Synthetic preservatives such as BHA and BHT are then added to preserve the oil; and the oils are subjected to great heat and are hydrogenated, denuding them of much of their life force.

Try to obtain oils that have no preservatives and are unhydrogenated and unheated. You can usually find these in special sections of supermarkets and at health food stores. There is much data to show that these wonderful oils are protective against atherosclerosis.

Be sure to refrigerate these good oils after opening, as

they have little in the way of natural preservatives left over and can spoil quickly if not kept cool.

We can also obtain good oil from the ingestion of nuts and seeds. In addition to oil, they are also rich in essential minerals and are fairly good sources of protein. They are best eaten raw and unsalted, and they make great snacks.

What about getting our oils from margarine? After all, don't the labels indicate that they are made from "pure vegetable oils?" While it is true that margarines are made from corn oil, safflower oil, and other highly unsaturated oils, the question we must ask ourselves is, "If margarine is made of safflower oil (for example), why is it hard and not liquid?" The answer is that virtually all margarines have been at least partially saturated—partially hardened—by a process known as "hydrogenation." This involves changing a great deal of the pure vegetable oil from a vegetable fat— unsaturated—to a chemical very much like animal fat—saturated.

The authors feel that a better answer to margarine is something they call Better Butter. Better Butter begins with real butter—which is about forty percent unsaturated and is a natural food containing high amounts of vitamin A, trace amounts of other vitamins, and small amounts of important minerals. To the butter is added pure, unprocessed safflower oil, the most unsaturated of all the vegetable oils. Lecithin, one of nature's most natural emulsifiers and an enemy of cholesterol, is the final ingredient.

Better Butter
1 lb. butter
1 cup safflower oil
½ cup granular lecithin

Blend until smooth. Pour into containers and refrigerate or freeze.

Better Butter contains nothing processed or artificial. It feels, tastes, and spreads like butter. It can be used wherever butter is used, and it is so much better for you.

The Case for Foods

So, there they are—the first three of the five nutritional essentials of cellular health. Good nutrition begins with good food. If you believe in the universal life force dwelling in your body, you should believe that it is good foods which potentiate this life force. Food is a holy communion between God and our cells. Do not think we can eat poorly and then supplement our diets with minerals and vitamins to sustain and improve health. A bad diet with supplements is still a bad diet! Do not think we can regularly eat harmful foods and affirm health. We must affirm by our actions. If our creed is health and wholeness, then our deeds must follow.

Not even Jesus would put the Lord to a foolish test. When the devil took Him up to the pinnacle of the temple and told Him to throw Himself down because if He really were the Son of God the angels " '. . . *will bear you up, lest you strike your foot against a stone.*' " Jesus said: " . . . *'You shall not tempt the Lord your God.*' " (Luke 4:11, 12)

And what do we do when we knowingly eat harmful foods and drink harmful beverages? Are we not putting God to a foolish test by brazenly disobeying His physical laws and then asking Him to save us? When we are faced with a harmful food, we must do as Jesus did. When He was tempted by the devil, He said: " . . . *'You shall worship the Lord your God, and him only shall you serve.*' " (Luke 4:8) We must say: *I worship the life force in me and that only shall I serve.*

25

Supplements Are Affirmations

Before beginning a discussion of vitamins and minerals, a short digression is in order. Those of us who write and lecture about health hardly ever get an argument when speaking of the correlation between eating properly and good health. Most people recognize the fact that good food is fundamental to their feeling of well-being. We get into trouble sometimes, however, when we mention vitamin and mineral supplementation. The arguments usually go something like this: "If God wanted us to have so many vitamins, He would have put them in our food." Or, "I eat a balanced diet, so I get enough vitamins."

While it is true that God did not give us vitamins and minerals in pill form, neither did He give us wings, wheels, or propellers. We were, however, given the intellect to discover wings so that we can "fly" higher than birds, to discover wheels so the we can "run" faster than horses, to discover propellers so that we can "swim" faster than fish. We were also given the intellect to discover food supplements so that we can "eat" better than all these animals.

As for the "balanced diet" argument, there is a basic flaw in its logic. In order for a food to be perfect, it must have been raised on perfect soil with optimum amounts of soil nutrients, sun, and rain. It would have to have been picked at the peak of its maturity. After harvest it would have to have been sustained at that maturity until we ate it.

Realizing the fact that nutrients are altered and destroyed by storage, cooking, and even sunlight, it is logical to assume that few if any foods are optimum when we eat them.

Look outside your window at the vegetation around you. The trees must compete with other trees for water. The grass competes also, taking some of the nutrients that

26

the trees would use; and flowers take their share, as do the weeds. In short, all these things have to be satisfied with less than perfect nutrition because they are stationary organisms and have no way of improving their own environment.

We, however, are different. We can improve our environment and our nutrition.

Adding vitamin and mineral supplements to our regular diet should be equated with adding affirmations to our regular thinking. When we want to prevent an occurrence in or change an aspect of our life, we begin by denying that which is not true about the situation and constantly affirming that which is for our highest benefit.

So it is with vitamin and mineral supplementation. If we feel we need help with a physical situation, we "deny" ourselves the harmful foods and "affirm" beneficial nutrients in the form of good foods and supplements.

If we want to do the best for our bodies, we will give them what they need. If we feel our diet is not adequate for our life-style, we should feel free to add vitamin and mineral supplements to it. Vitamins and minerals potentiate the life force in the body; but remember, they can only do so in the presence of positive thoughts and good foods.

Now that we know that good nutrition begins with good foods, and we know what the good foods are, let's turn to an essential that appears in all good foods (albeit not always in optimum amounts). This essential is an organic substance that is necessary in tiny amounts to control our metabolic processes. It cannot be synthesized by the body; therefore, it must be obtained from our diet. We are speaking, of course, of vitamins. The importance of vitamins is indicated by the first four letters of the word itself. *Vita* means "life."

Vitamins are truly "small wonders." They perform their life-giving feats in the body in amounts that are not measured in pounds or even ounces, but in grams (one twenty-seventh of an ounce), milligrams (one thousandth of a gram), and micrograms (one millionth of a gram!). God shows His grandeur as much in His use of vitamins to control the metabolic processes in each cell as He does in controlling the orbits of all the planets and stars.

Charles Fillmore talked about . . . *the invisible life elements that physical science has named vitamins.* And they *are* invisible to us. But our little factories of life—our cells—recognize these vitamins and hungrily appropriate them into their inner sanctum where, with the other essentials, the cells busily distill their only product—life.

Vitamins are generally divided into two categories. The first is the fat-soluble vitamins which are found in foods containing fat and are absorbed only with dietary fat. The fat-soluble vitamins are vitamins A, D, E, and K. Since they are absorbed with fat, conditions unfavorable to fat absorption would create a deficiency of these vitamins. Because there is no quick way for the body to get rid of the fat-soluble vitamins, they are easily stored in the body and we are not necessarily dependent on a day-to-day supply.

The second category is the water-soluble vitamins. These are, as the name would imply, soluble in water. Thus, they are excreted in small amounts in the urine and cannot be stored in the body. The water-soluble vitamins are vitamin C and the vitamins of the B complex. We cannot make or store these vitamins, so the body is dependent upon a day-to-day source in the form of the foods we eat or the supplements we take.

Each vitamin has its own area of influence—of expertise. Thus, vitamin A is essential to the health of the skin, eyes, and mucous membranes lining the mouth, the digestive, respiratory, and genitourinary tracts. It even influences the development of the teeth!

The only food sources of vitamin A are animal sources, such as liver, whole milk, and eggs. (There are others.) However, the body can convert the carotene in many plants to vitamin A. Such plant sources include carrots, squashes, sweet potatoes, and many other yellow and green plants.

Vitamin E, on the other hand, works on our behalf a bit more subtly. As the powerful antioxidant, Vitamin E prevents the oxidation of unsaturated molecules, which many believe leads to premature aging. It is a potent inhibitor of blood clotting and is important in preventing and ameliorating any cardiovascular and peripheral vascular diseases.

A good food source of vitamin E is high quality vegetable oils, especially wheat germ oil. However, many scientists believe it is extremely difficult to obtain enough vitamin E from the diet alone and that supplementation is advisable.

Vitamin D is essential if we are to absorb calcium and, to some extent, phosphorus. Without vitamin D in our bodies, all the calcium we ingest is excreted. (Without sufficient calcium, bones become brittle and easily breakable.) Vitamin D has been called the "sunshine vitamin" because it is possible for the body to utilize the ultraviolet light from the sun to make it. Saltwater fish is another good source of vitamin D (including cod liver oil), as are liver and eggs.

Vitamin K is needed for the normal function of the liver and for normal blood clotting. Good sources are: most green leafy vegetables, tomatoes, eggs, and liver.

Vitamin K is one of the few vitamins the body can make itself. It is synthesized by the intestinal flora, which, if the intestinal area is kept relatively healthy, should always produce enough to prevent a frank deficiency.

Because the B complex and vitamin C are water-soluble, it is important to realize that they can easily be destroyed by cooking. This is especially true when foods rich in these vitamins are cooked for long periods of time in a lot of water and the water is then discarded. In order to protect the water-soluble vitamins, it is best, instead of boiling foods, to steam them for as short a period as possible.

B complex—There are eleven members of the B complex family, and we need all of them. The B vitamins are the spark plugs of the body. Without them, nothing else works. They are responsible for the metabolism of our nutrients. They give us energy and good nerves. But remember, the B vitamins are a complex. They work together as a team. If one or more is missing from our diet, the team does not function properly, and ultimately, we fail.

The following are the generally accepted vitamins of the B complex: B1 (thiamine), B2 (riboflavin), Niacin (or niacinamide), Pantothenic acid, PABA (Para Aminobenzoic acid), B6 (pyridoxine), B12, Folic acid, Biotin, Choline, and Inositol.

The best sources of all the B complex are organ meats (especially liver), whole grains and cereals (especially wheat germ), yeast (brewer's type, *not* live yeast), eggs, dark green leafy vegetables, and some legumes.

Metabolism does not begin without the B complex, nor does it proceed smoothly with insufficient amounts. Since they are important in the body's handling of stress, be sure you are adequately supplied with this key family of nutrients—especially if your life-style is one filled with stress.

Vitamin C—It is difficult to write about vitamin C without making it sound like a superstar; it is essential for such a multitude of metabolic processes. It is needed if we are to break down our protein properly. It is also needed for red blood cell development—the key to an abundant energy level. Broken bones or wounded tissues do not mend without vitamin C. Iron is not absorbed without vitamin C. Vitamin C enhances our capacity to withstand injury from burns and bacterial toxins. It is most important in times of stress. It has been shown effective in preventing the common cold and is essential to the formation of collagen—the "cement" that holds the cells together. Vitamin C does all of this and much, much more.

We are one of the few animals on Earth who can't synthesize our own vitamin C. And, because we cannot store it, we are dependent on the day-to-day supply contained in the foods we eat.

Some good food sources of vitamin C are: guava, parsley, turnip greens, peppers, broccoli, cabbage, strawberries, and citrus fruits.

Be sure this superstar appears in your diet, and don't be afraid to take it as a supplement if it does not.

Minerals Reflect Our Oneness

No nutritional essential reflects our oneness with the Earth and the universe as do minerals, or elements. A look at the Periodic Table of Elements in any chemistry book shows that there are currently 103 known elements. These elements or minerals are the same whether they are present in the stars, the Earth, or in the body! And minerals are as essential to life as are vitamins, fats, carbohydrates, and protein.

Because minerals are inorganic, plants and animals cannot create them. The plants obtain their minerals from the soil, and the animals must obtain their minerals from the plants or other animals that eat the plants. (It is obvious what happens when our soil is deficient in minerals to begin with, isn't it?)

Because they are inorganic, minerals are not "burned up" by the body. This, of course, does not mean that they are not "used up." They are, and they must be replaced. They are excreted from the body in the perspiration, the feces, and especially the urine.

As with vitamins and the other essentials, a deficiency in a mineral will manifest itself as a challenge to our health. Goiter, rickets, and anemia are but a few of these manifestations. However, an important thing to remember is that, just as there is an interrelationship and must be a balance between the three phases of man, there is a relationship and balance necessary between the five nutritional essentials. Minerals, like vitamins, fats, carbohydrates, and proteins, are dependent on other nutrients and other minerals for their proper functioning. The minerals are interrelated and balanced with each other in human chemistry. Without one, the others depending on it would not function properly. For example, cobalt, iron, and copper are all essential to the formation of red blood cells. And calcium and phosphorus are in a crucial relationship in the formation of teeth and bones.

Minerals also work with vitamins. For example, magnesium and vitamin B6 work together, as do calcium and vitamin D.

Vitamins are not the only nutrients that need minerals in order to work properly. The mineral phosphorus, for instance, plays an essential role in the proper metabolism of carbohydrates, proteins, and fats. It is also important for nervous tissue metabolism and skeletal growth. The mineral zinc is necessary for the building of protein. Fat and sugar metabolism depend on chromium. In short, minerals are an integral part of any complete program of health. Because we don't hear as much about minerals as we do vitamins does not lessen their importance.

Minerals are usually classified as "major" minerals and "trace" minerals. The major minerals are calcium, phosphorus, magnesium, sodium, potassium, sulfur, chlorine, and silicon.

The trace minerals are iron, manganese, chromium, zinc, copper, cobalt, molybdenum, fluorine, iodine, selenium, and vanadium.

If our diet is poor, it is a safe bet that we are deficient in minerals. An optimum diet—that is, eating the five essentials in addition to a liberal amount of raw, unsalted nuts and seeds—would go a long way toward fulfilling the body's needs for minerals.

If you feel you need more minerals than you are getting in your food, don't deny the life force in your cells the raw materials it needs to build health. Supplement your food intake. Some good supplemental sources of minerals that are available in powder or tablet form are: kelp—which, being a sea plant, contains virtually all the trace minerals; also rich in trace minerals is alfalfa (tablets made from the juice of the alfalfa plant are excellent); bone meal is another fine source of all the minerals, especially calcium; or you may find a multi-mineral tablet to your liking available at your local health food store.

An important point to remember is that minerals are not single elements working alone. The body needs many in its quest for the holy grail of life. It is our sacred duty to recognize this need and to present the body with the raw materials necessary for its continued health and wholeness.

That completes our discussion of the five essentials for cellular life—primary protein, constructive carbohydrates, fundamental fatty acids (oils), mandatory minerals, and vital vitamins. We need them all. Getting only some of them is like trying to drive a car with only some of the spark plugs. We can do it for a while, but ultimately we will fail.

(Did you remember to mark this section for later reference?)

Health is a commitment. *Total* health is a *total* commitment. A commitment to good nutrition *alone* is not enough.

We will have short, sad lives indeed unless we use these five essentials in conjunction with regular exercise, adequate rest, and abundant fresh air and sunshine. And all these are utterly useless unless they are supplemental to thoughts of God, of life, of health, and of wholeness. Charles Fillmore said: *When the chemistry of the body and the dynamics of the mind are united, a third element is brought forth, and man feels that "in Christ, he is a new creature."*

Vegetarian—To Be or Not To Be

There are probably very few of us in the Truth movement who have not at some time at least considered the possibility of becoming vegetarians. Those of us in the Unity movement are aware of the Fillmores' viewpoint on the subject and of the support vegetarianism has been given through the succeeding decades.

Charles and Myrtle Fillmore were staunch vegetarians for many years and were strong in their desire that others in Unity do likewise. Thomas Witherspoon, in his informative and entertaining book, *Myrtle Fillmore: Mother of Unity*, relates the following story: . . . *on one occasion he* [Charles Fillmore] *came upon a worker about to bite into a hot dog, and with much fanfare and laughter, he ceremoniously nailed the bit of meat to a tree.*

During the 1920s the Unity Vegetarian Inn was one of the most popular eating places in Kansas City. While that restaurant has long since vanished, the tradition of vegetarianism in Unity has carried over to the present-day Inn at Unity Village, where, although meat is served, a meatless entrée is offered at each meal.

Because the idea of vegetarianism is so confusing to many people, it might be a good idea to actually define the term and then to objectively examine aspects on both sides of the issue. In this way you can make up your own mind as to which path to follow.

The first thing we must realize of course is that each of us *is* a temple of God and that our duty lies in the proper care of this temple. The eighteenth statement of "Unity's

Statement of Faith" declares: *We believe that the body of man is the highest-formed manifestation of creative Mind and that it is capable of unlimited expression of that Mind. "Know ye not that your body is a temple of the Holy Spirit?"*

The responsibility to this temple is a vast and vital one. We are *the highest-formed manifestation of the creative Mind;* but this implies an inherent responsibility—one that cannot be shirked if we are to let our unlimited capabilities unfold. God's physical laws are to be learned and obeyed. Maintaining the body temple is a continual project that must not be treated lightly. There is no room for apathy or complacency. We cannot afford to coast. When we are coasting, there is one thing we can be sure of: we are going downhill!

No, coasting will never bring us perfection. If we avow that we are God's temple, if we believe we have a God-given *right* to enjoy health, then we must realize that we have a God-given *responsibility* to maintain health.

Myrtle Fillmore once said: *We must know the chemistry of the body. We must feed the whole man. We have to have this outer man and have to make the mortar that builds him up. . . . Your first duty is to bless your body. Get your thoughts right down into it, and praise its wonderful work. Learn what it needs and arrange for supplying those needs.* She was absolutely right! We must first learn the body's needs and then supply those needs.

That Myrtle was so very aware of the necessity of proper nutrition is evidenced by a letter to the famous nutritionist Dr. Bengamin Gayelord Hauser. In her later years her own health was not what it might have been, and so in 1930 she wrote to Hauser for help: *There will come a time when we can draw forth the universal mind stuff, just the elements we need in the right proportion and relation, to maintain the proper balance in our organisms. We shall be able to draw chemical substances from the fourth dimensional realm, down into our physical body. But in the meantime, we need to make practical all the knowledge we have concerning bodily renewal, through using intelligence and discrimination in the selection of our food. And so I am asking your help, and shall be glad for anything that you can tell me, to help along the work of bodily transformation and renewal.*

She was never able to get to New York to work with Dr. Hauser. If she had, one can only speculate as to what new or different ideas the Fillmores might have adopted in their nutrition regime. Charles always said he reserved the right to change his mind. He was a man of scientific thinking, always in the *avant garde* on new issues. It is safe to assume that he would be most receptive to all the latest scientific data concerning the nutritional needs of the body temple were he alive today.

The question for us, then, is not so much whether we should become or remain vegetarians. The important question is: How can we best nourish our body temples? Vegetarian or non-vegetarian, it is possible to become malnourished or well-nourished following either course.

That is why, after Myrtle met Dr. Hauser in 1928 when he was speaking in Kansas City, she was so impressed by his words: *How is Unity going to build those new buildings at the farm—by thinking them only? No, indeed, you are getting the very best building materials and placing them together according to the blueprints. And we must get the very best materials, suited to the body's needs, and place them together according to the blueprints of our health and perfect bodies.*

This made good sense to Myrtle then and it makes good sense to us today. With all this in mind, let us now look at exactly what vegetarianism is.

Varieties of Vegetarians

There are three types of vegetarians. The first are those we call lacto-ovo-vegetarians, who eat no animal flesh but do eat eggs, milk, and milk products. The second group is called lacto-vegetarian because from animal sources they consume only milk and milk products. The third group is that which consumes no animal products whatsoever, eating only fruits, vegetables, nuts, seeds, and grain. These people are often referred to as fruitarians or vegans.

So you can see that within the parameters of vegetarianism there is a wide scope, with many choices to be made. It is not the intention of this chapter to advise you in what ultimately must be your own decision nor to make a judgment as to which path is "better." But it is the intention of this chapter to present enough spiritual and scientific considerations to enable you to make up your own mind. We will begin where we should always begin—with the spiritual.

Spiritual Considerations

It has often been said that one becomes more spiritual after giving up meat. This is not necessarily true. In fact, it is more likely that, if anything, the opposite is true—as one becomes more spiritual, one may want to give up meat! There is a Unity pamphlet entitled "Vegetarianism" which quotes Charles Fillmore: *You must recognize that there is but one universal life, one universal substance, one universal intelligence, and that every animal is contending for its life and is entitled to that life.*

The pamphlet then goes on to say that *there is a kindred spirit in all living things, a love for life. Any man who considers honestly the oneness of life feels an aversion to eating meat that is a natural reaction of his mind toward anything so foreign to the idea of universal life, love, and freedom.* Good point, well-stated. The idea of our oneness with all life is certainly a valid and loving motivation for vegetarianism in the minds of many.

This pamphlet goes even further as it states: *We believe wholeheartedly that the time will come when the race will have so accepted vegetarianism that it will look back upon meat eating with the same aversion that it now looks upon cannibalism, and all life will be sacred.* Too strong a statement? Not necessarily. These are issues we must each face because, as the same pamphlet reflects: *As he develops spiritually, man comes to question seriously the rightness of meat as a part of his diet.*

Myrtle's philosophy of "no murdered thing" was well known, and it prompted her to be a vegetarian for the last thirty-six years of her life. Charles followed the same path, although he did begin to eat fish in his last years. (Remember that he always reserved the right to change his mind!) But his writings contain many strong arguments against flesh foods. He once predicted: *New and better foods will be found to replace the corrupt flesh with which people have been stuffing their stomachs.*

There is ample argument, from a spiritual viewpoint, to support the decision to become a vegetarian. But, as always, we can find support for the opposite side too. The Bible is full of such support. There are numerous references to the eating of meat. We are told that man is given dominion over all things—that everything is here for our purpose.

Jesus is depicted as a meat eater. *For I was an hungered, and ye gave me meat.* (Matt. 25:35 A.V.) And after the Resurrection, when He appeared to His disciples, He ate fish. In Luke 24:41-43 A.V., we read: *. . . he said unto them, Have ye here any meat? And they gave him a piece of broiled fish, and of an honeycomb. And he took* it, *and did eat before them.*

Whether this incident had anything to do with Charles Fillmore's decision to eat fish, we do not know. But there are many advanced metaphysicians who interpret this Bible passage as meaning there is something in fish that is needed by the perfect body form. This, certainly, is an interpretation that is subject to individual acceptance. It is included here because it points up the fact that there is no easy answer to the question of flesh eating, even among the most spiritual Truth students.

Your own decision as to what is best for you can only be reached after much meditation and seeking.

The Scientific Side

Now, what if you decide vegetarianism is right for you? What does science have to say in the matter? It is time to examine carefully the nutritional aspects of the issue so that you can make an intelligent evaluation of your body temple's needs, keeping in mind that we must always work with God's laws which govern that temple.

The chief building material of the body temple is protein, so it follows that good protein—in adequate amounts—is our first nutritional requirement. And where do we get protein? We get the best protein from eggs, milk and milk products, lean meat, fish, and poultry. There is some protein in grains, nuts, seeds, fruits, and vegetables; but it is generally incomplete or unbalanced in amino acids and therefore inefficiently utilized by the body as protein when eaten alone.

The fact is that the top-grade, complete (containing the eight essential amino acids in a proper balance) protein can be obtained only from the animal or its products. (The amino acid content of foods can be found in many government and scientific publications.)

What this means is that grains, nuts, seeds, fruits, and vegetables, though they are fine foods, cannot be relied upon as main sources of protein if eaten alone. It would be analagous to building a house of straw instead of brick and stone.

If, however, you choose to keep all animal products out of your diet, you must be extremely careful to combine your other foods so that they complement each other in amino acid content and balance.

Put as simply as possible, we need protein because of the amino acids it contains. These amino acids are the "building blocks" of protein. There are a certain amount and a certain balance of amino acids that are critical. Eggs, milk and milk products, cheese, fish, fowl, and meat are called "top-grade" proteins because they contain the proper amounts of amino acids in the proper balance; thus, even when eaten alone, they are complete proteins.

Grains, nuts, seeds, fruits, and vegetables, while they do contain amino acids, generally do not contain them in either the right amounts or in the proper balance. However, it is possible, if you are skillful, to combine these foods so that the amino acid strength of one food will supplement the amino acid weakness of another food, thereby in combination making a finer protein food than either food separately.

For instance, legumes (peas, beans, etc.) are deficient in an essential amino acid called methionine. Without this essential amino acid, legumes are an inferior protein source and will not build healthy human tissue. Grains are also deficient in an essential amino acid, this one is called lysine. Because of this deficiency they, too, are an inferior protein and will not build the most healthy human tissue. However, it just so happens that legumes, while being low in methionine, are high in lysine. Grains, on the other hand, while being low in lysine, are high in methionine. When these two foods—legumes and grains—are combined at the same meal they supplement each other's weaknesses and form a much superior protein capable of building much more superior tissue than either alone. Some common examples of this type of combining include beans and rice, corn bread and black-eyed peas, even peanut butter on whole grain bread! Eaten alone, legumes and grains are incomplete and, therefore, inferior protein foods. However, when combined, they are complete.

If you are going to eat this way, shunning all animal protein, it is essential that you make a thorough study and learn how to combine your foods. (There are several books written for the layman that can help you.)

We must recognize that there are not many separate laws; there is only one law—God's law. And chemistry and the science of nutrition are simply one facet of God's law. Who else but the divine Creator planned and built it all? So it is important to keep in mind that the laws by which our bodies function are part of the divine design and cannot be tampered with or ignored if we wish to do the will of God and maintain His holy temple.

Therefore, if we were fashioned out of protein and require it for all repair, maintenance, and regeneration of the body, it behooves us to cooperate with the life force within us and work according to the blueprint of our being.

The importance of protein is of such magnitude that it cannot possibly be emphasized enough. As we have seen, however, it is not necessary to eat flesh foods in order to obtain top-grade, complete protein. If your decision is to avoid meats, you can be perfectly healthy by using eggs, or milk and milk products, or all three. In fact, the egg is the most perfect source of protein that exists. (The undue concern about the cholesterol content of the egg is finally being

mollified by more recent studies which seem to indict the refined carbohydrates, especially sugar and white flour, as the
culprits in raising serum cholesterol.)

By eating milk, milk products (unprocessed cheese and
cottage cheese, yogurt, etc.), and/or eggs, you can obtain
superior nutrition without taking life. (The eggs from com-
mercial producers are not fertile.) Thus, you are a vegetarian who is giving himself the best nutrition according to
science. Remember, if you choose to be a vegan—one who
eats nothing from an animal—be sure you know how to
combine your foods to yield the highest protein possible.

We should be interested enough in our body temples
to want to investigate exactly what is scientific and what is
not. God works through science, and it is important for us
to know our needs and how to supply them.

The Vitamin B12 Trap

There is an aspect of vegetarianism of which we should
be aware, and that is our body's need for vitamin B12. This
essential vitamin factor is available only in animal products.
Its deficiency will cause pernicious anemia. If you are going
to eat *no* animal food (not only no flesh foods, but no eggs
and milk products as well), it is essential that you supplement your diet with some vitamin B12.

There is a trap into which strict vegans can easily fall,
and that is a hidden B12 deficiency. People who eat a lot of
green leafy vegetables are getting an abundance of another
B complex vitamin, folic acid, in their diets. Folic acid can
mask a vitamin B12 deficiency and so for many years a
severe B12 lack can go undetected. Eventually it makes itself known, and at that point it is a very serious state of
affairs.

So be certain to take a vitamin B12 tablet regularly if

you are not eating any animal products. The body cannot live without it since it is part of our divine design.

A Word About Soybeans

Many vegetarians, especially vegans, rely very heavily on soybeans as their main source of protein. However, raw soybeans have some undesirable factors that are harmful to the human body. Heating soybeans destroys most but not all of these factors, making it a better food but still not a great food. When soybeans are prepared, therefore, it is wise to thoroughly wash them and then cook or steam them. It may be even wiser, however, to use soybeans more sparingly in your diet and rely instead on all the other fine foods available. As was mentioned earlier, nuts, seeds, grains, fruits, and vegetables are fine foods when eaten alone and can be combined to yield a good grade of protein.

Finding Our Path

The decision as to what path to follow is an important and a difficult one, as you can see. It requires much prayerful reflection as well as scientific investigation. The main thing is to recognize the body as the temple of the Holy Spirit, and when we do, we will make the right decision because we will want to do the very best for it. We will come to know what Charles Fillmore realized when he wrote: . . . *we have endeavored to reconcile a dying body with a living God, but have not succeeded.*

God is indeed God of the living. Our temple must reflect life and vibrancy. *The time is ripe for the advent of a new race, the advent of the spiritualized man. This will be brought about, not by a miracle or the fiat of God, but by the gradual refinement of the man of the flesh into the man of the Spirit,* said Charles Fillmore.

Religious dedication to careful selection of our food is an essential factor in helping to bring about this *new race.* Our tissues must be refined and strengthened with the very finest foods. This is what Mr. Fillmore was telling us when he wrote: *There is a relationship between thinking and eating, and as you grow spiritually the character of your food and all that pertains to eating may have to be changed in conformity with the new order of things.*

The more we develop our unlimited spiritual potential the more we will be guided to perfect the body temple that houses that Spirit. Whatever our decision about vegetarianism at this time, let us eat with thanksgiving, blessing the wonderful nutrients we are building into our temples, and knowing that the creative force within us will utilize them properly and efficiently.

Thank You, Father, for life and the good food to nourish that life.

Fatigue

There is enough energy within one human being to run an entire city! To many of us that fact, scientific as it may be, would seem almost laughable. "Me? Power a city? Why, I can hardly drag myself through the day," might be the response. It seems that the most common complaint of people when it comes to their physical states is that of lack of energy—chronic fatigue. Some of us are tired before we ever get out of bed in the morning. It is an effort to go to work, an effort to care for the house, and even an effort to pray. We are just too tired. And, when we are perpetually tired, life loses much of its meaning as we lumber from day to day discouraged and apathetic.

If this describes you, you will be happy to learn the good news: *It doesn't have to be that way!* That's right. There are thoughts you can think and things you can do that can change your life from one of listlessness to one of liveliness. It's true! You probably feel better already just knowing there is a way out of your lethargy—a way others have successfully taken and which you, if you sincerely desire to, can take as well.

There are three basic steps to overcoming fatigue. Do you have enough energy to read on? Yes? Good. The first step can be taken sitting or even lying down. That's even more good news, isn't it! So get comfortable, put your feet up, and let's begin.

Your Body of Lights

Your body is a body of light. Jesus told us this almost 2,000 years ago. But it wasn't until recently that scientists had seen the evidence of it. What they discovered was that at the center of every atom there is light. In fact, all matter is energy, and some scientists are speculating that this energy is basically light.

Now that is exciting! Your body is truly made up of trillions of tiny lights, all sparkling and twinkling and flashing with a glittering array of myriad colors. Picture it. Stop reading for a moment, put the book down, and close your eyes. Begin to see the dazzling spectacle of your own being. Breathe deeply, sensing the vibrations of all of those trillions of lights as they glow within your cells. Feel the currents of energy that this brilliance generates as it beams itself through your entire being and then radiates outward into the universe.

You are one with the universe. The lights come and go in the eternal ethers, gliding in and out of your being in an infinite exchange of energy. You are never the same as the moment before—always new, always reborn. Become aware of the continual flow of this stream of universal energy as it passes through your body. Realize that the Source is unlimited, unending, and undefatigable. The energy is *always* there.

What is *not* always there is our awareness of it or our cooperation with it. *Modern science tells us that in the trillions of cells in our body there are imprisoned electronic energies beyond all possibility of estimate; that a single teardrop has within its atoms dynamic force enough to blow up a six-story building. Man is coming into an understanding of how to release these mighty powers and use them in regenerating soul and body. Charles Fillmore was most enthu-*

47

siastic about the atom-smashing power within each of us.

We know that when Jesus healed people He was releasing the latent energy within their cells. In other words, the energy of the life force is there all the time—it is always within us and available to us.

Focus Your Energies

Much of the time we scatter our energies. We can use them for constructive or destructive purposes. It is up to us. If we do not engage in daily prayer and meditation in order to attune ourselves with the Christ Mind within us, we find that our energies are dissipated into meaningless and frenzied activities. Unless we endeavor to remain centered in the Christ, seeking first the kingdom of God in all situations, we are apt to be faced with a feeling of frustration and fatigue.

When we pray and meditate we release large amounts of energy that has been lying dormant in the cells. This energy has an effect on the physical body and helps to generate and invigorate it.

Every thought we think radiates an energy as it passes through the nervous system. Strong, positive thoughts create positive, constructive energy. The opposite is true of negative thoughts—they will tear us down as surely and systematically as a long illness. That is why we must never say we are weak or tired or sick or old. The body temple is constructed according to laws that are *always* in effect. According to these laws it is the duty of our body cells to cooperate with what we believe and decree. If we are thinking and decreeing weakness, then it must follow that weakness is what we will get.

Work with Twelve Powers

It might be interesting to work with some of the twelve powers of man in your attempt to fight fatigue. Strength would be an obvious faculty on which to concentrate. Strength is really the idea of endurance. Always affirm: *I am strength.* (This is much more effective than saying, "I have strength.") *I am strength!* Repeat it often during the day, silently as well as audibly.

The body center for the strength faculty lies in the back, in the area of the adrenal glands. It would seem to be more than coincidence that the adrenals are responsible for releasing adrenalin—so essential in helping to regulate the body's fuel and therefore its energy. The adrenals are also involved in hypoglycemia (low blood sugar), and hypoglycemia is very often a chief factor in chronic fatigue.

Another power that seems appropriate to work with is zeal. Here is our inner fire—the ability to achieve something with enthusiasm and success. We can use this faculty to its best advantage in a spiritual way, letting it give us the energy and the desire to unlock our true potential as we strive to maintain our sense of oneness with the universal life force. *In the human body spiritual zeal, that is, enthusiasm, electrifies the nerve substance, which breaks forth into energy,* declared Mr. Fillmore, who once made the remark: *I fairly sizzle with zeal . . . .*

As you can see, there is much one can do, working in the spiritual realm, to activate new energies in the body temple. Eventually you can build a state of consciousness that excludes all thoughts and suggestions of negativism, weakness, and fatigue. This takes persistence, but it can be done. Then you will continually think of yourself as a body of shimmering colors of light. And much of this can be practiced while lying down!

Exercise Builds Strength

It is time now, however, to get onto your feet as we move to Step Two of our program. Believe it or not, physical exercise gives us energy if done correctly and regularly. In fact, the less active you become the more tired you become. You can prove this for yourself—but you'll have to exercise to do so!

A nice brisk walk is good exercise. Try that. Or try some swimming or cycling or yoga or mild calisthenics. You will have to find the exercise that works best for you. There are plenty of good ones. To begin with you won't want to do too much. But, as your nutrition improves, it is remarkable how soon you will find new strength coming into your muscles when you exercise regularly. Physical exercise is one of the three steps in our fatigue-fighting program. Each step is important and must be practiced. So, move the muscles, blessing them for their wonderful strength. Enjoy your exercise, knowing how the life force rejoices in constructive motion.

Foods Fight Fatigue

We are ready at this point to move into our third step, that of proper nutrition. It is time to examine what we have been using for the building materials for the body temple because a good part of the blame for tiredness often lies in the food we eat. Let's check it out.

Are you eating enough top-grade protein? The hemoglobin molecule, the iron-containing pigment of the red blood cell so essential for energy, is built mostly of protein. Only a small percentage of it is iron. This means that an inadequate supply of protein can result in poverty-stricken blood. This could be a big part of your answer. We *must* have protein. Does each of your meals—and snacks—include at least one of the primary proteins? (Now is the time to refer back to that all-important section you have specially marked on page 17.)

Are you eating the constructive carbohydrates that provide the right fuel for the body? (See page 20)

And are you making sure that some good vegetable oil is included in your diet? Use one that is mechanically pressed and unpreserved, but do refrigerate it after opening. These oils are sold in health stores and are well worth the few extra pennies. (See page 22)

Begin with Breakfast

Do you eat breakfast? This is a key consideration because those who do not eat breakfast are the ones most likely to experience chronic fatigue. Breakfast is the most important meal of the day.

If you do eat breakfast, what kind do you eat? The life force residing in your cells does not consider coffee and a bun to be an acceptable breakfast. By good breakfast we mean some protein and a constructive carbohydrate. There are all kinds of breakfasts that can be considered good. Most people would select eggs, toast, milk, and a piece of fruit. This is excellent. But so would be cottage cheese and fresh fruit, or a lean ground beef patty on a whole grain bun with a glass of milk, or a cheese omelet and a piece of toast. The possibilities are vast. But it must be based on one of the top-grade sources of protein in order for it to qualify for a good breakfast. Whole grain cereals (such as oatmeal or granola) are fine to use but should be counted as a carbohydrate source, not a protein source.

A good breakfast determines the energy level for the day. If you don't want to *eat* a breakfast, how about *drink-*

ing one? A delicious and energizing drink can be made in the blender and then sipped at breakfast time. Here is a typical recipe. Blend the following:

8 ounces non-fat milk
1 or 2 raw eggs
1 tablespoonful protein powder (milk and egg type is best)
½ teaspoonful of wheat germ oil
½ banana (or other small piece of fruit or some honey)

This is a power-packed drink and should be sipped *very slowly.* Try it and see what a difference it can make in the way you feel.

Hypoglycemia was mentioned earlier as a possible cause of fatigue. If you suspect this might be the case, be sure to eat many small meals a day—each with a good protein source—and keep away from the junk foods and refined carbohydrates. (For more information on hypoglycemia you can refer to the chapter titled "High Hopes for Hypoglycemia."

Don't Overlook Supplements

You will feel better if you take some supplements. A complete, high-potency multiple vitamin supplement, one that is very high in the total B complex (eleven B vitamins), is good as a basis. Then try adding some extra vitamin C. (Less than 3,000 milligrams per day will probably be ineffective.) Vitamin C helps fight fatigue. It enhances the absorption of iron and is necessary for the proper utilization of several B complex vitamins.

You might next try adding an iron supplement. Read your label and try to purchase one that says ferrous (iron) gluconate, fumerate, peptonate, or citrate. Or use the chelated (pronounced kee-lated) iron. Many find that these forms work best and all of them are well received by the body.

All of the above will help to nourish your tissues, giving them the raw materials they crave. Remember, however, that good nutrition begins with a good breakfast.

Liver, Liver, Liver

There is one special food that can be of enormous help to anyone suffering from chronic or even temporary fatigue. That food is liver. Eat liver as often as possible and on the days when you don't eat it, take desiccated liver tablets or capsules. If you use the tablets (or capsules) you will have to take them by the handsful because you will want to take the equivalent of a serving of liver. Ten or fifteen a day may be a good amount to begin with.

In addition to its high content of B vitamins—especially B12—liver has an as-yet-unisolated anti-fatigue factor. Many people have found liver to bring about a dramatic change in their energy levels. Several tablets in the mid-afternoon, along with a small glass of milk or tomato juice, may not exactly be gourmet fare but it is manna to the body temple. Try it and see if you don't agree.

Divine Transfusion

Finally, consider this. When the body gets too run-down, physicians often suggest a blood transfusion. Jesus came into the world to give the human race a "divine trans-fusion." His energy and love are everywhere around us, pervading our atmosphere, at all times available to us. We can make contact with this divine energy. We can appropri-ate it into our bodies and souls, letting it lift us and strengthen us and preserve us. We need proper exercise. We need good nutrition. But these in themselves, while necessary to the plan, are not enough. We need that "divine transfusion" that only our contact with the Christ can give.

Charles Fillmore expressed it in these words: *Men are to be alive — not merely exist half-dead for a few years and then go out with a sputter, like a tallow dip. Jesus Christ's men are to be electric lights that glow with a perpetual current from the one omnipresent Energy.*

We were created as divine creatures of light. If you have been hiding your light under the bushel basket of fatigue, you no longer need to do this. Take the three steps of the fatigue-fighting program and let your light shine from now on.

When we begin to let our whole being radiate with light, we give the life force the opportunity it eternally seeks—we become like those of whom the prophet Isaiah spoke: . . . *they who wait for the Lord shall renew their strength, they shall mount up with wings like eagles, they shall run and not be weary, they shall walk and not faint.* (Isa. 40:31) Will you settle for that?

Abolish Arthritis

Arthritis is one of the oldest recorded diseases. Paleontologic specimens reveal that even in prehistoric days the great dinosaurs were affected by arthritis. The mummies of ancient Egypt show evidence of this condition, and there are references to it in the literature and records of all the many civilizations that have appeared since then.

The divine laws that govern the body temple do not change from century to century, which means that we are manifesting the same "dis-eases" today as our ancestors did aeons ago because of the same abuse and disregard for the laws. But we in Truth are fortunate in knowing that the answers lie within us and that disease must be conquered by the forces that already dwell in the body temple.

The word "arthritis" means literally "joint inflammation." The result is almost always pain and stiffness, with body movement becoming difficult and often limited.

Movement is basic to life. All living things move— whether it is slow turning of a flower toward the sun, the graceful gliding of a ballerina across a stage, or the spectacular dive of a hawk toward its prey. Movement is indigenous to life. Any inhibition of movement is an inhibition of life and should be corrected so that the full potential of life can be expressed.

Arthritis is just such an inhibitor of movement and is therefore an inhibitor of life. It is not a normal condition and must be corrected if we are to express the perfection that we are. Charles Fillmore tells us: *We know that health is the normal condition of man and that it is a condition true to his real being.*

The fact that an estimated twenty million Americans suffer from arthritis indicates that its cause is deep-seated in human nature and stems from an area in our human psyche that needs strengthening. Most metaphysicians agree that the area that needs the most attention is in human relationships—in a word, love.

An analysis of any joint in the body will show that it is at the junction of two bones. The joint allows the bones to move in opposition to each other without friction. It allows opposition without conflict—and that is a key word: *conflict.* Metaphysician and healer Dr. Cushing Smith, writing on arthritis says: *. . . there is but one basic mental cause and that is conflict . . . disagreements and clashing opinions between two or more people are represented in arthritis.* He goes on to say: *Older people develop arthritis in proportion to their stiffened attitudes toward others, their unwillingness to cooperate, or the tendency to grow more and more "set in their ways."*

Catherine Ponder concurs with this. She writes in "The Healing Secret of the Ages": *Continual criticism is believed to produce rheumatism. People who suffer disease in their "joints" are usually people who are "out of joint" in their thinking.*

But how, you may ask, can thoughts or feelings or words have an effect on bodies? The answer is: because thoughts, feelings, and words are things! They affect our body chemistry as much as do the foods we eat. Charles Fillmore was one of many who believed that. He wrote: *In spiritual understanding we know that all the forces in the body are directed by thought and that they work in a constructive or a destructive way, according to the character of the thought.* Our bodies feed on our words, whether they are silent or audible. What our minds dwell on, our bodies will manifest. *We express physically what we dwell on mentally.*

We can use this wonderful power of the mind to our advantage. We release healing and renewing power merely by speaking words of life, joy, and love. We can begin renewing ourselves by our spoken word. It is true that our bodies feed on our words. Then why do we not make our words those of life and joy and love? Why not give our bodies these wonderful thoughts as the food with which they can build themselves?

Clara Palmer in her Unity book *You Can Be Healed* tells us: *A creaking or painful joint can be so lubricated with the oil of joy that it will work perfectly, but you must let go of every unyielding, bigoted, or set thought that acts as a joy killer. . . . Joy is a perfect lubricant.*

Warmth Is Helpful

Heat is very soothing to painful joints. This may indicate a need for the pervasive warmth that only love can bring. Unity author Mary Katherine MacDougall tells us that: *Love can dissolve any hard deposits in joints, can loosen up joints, can flex muscles.* She goes on to say that we must bless our bodies and picture them perfect in form. Then we . . . *drink in love with every mouthful of liquid, we eat love with every bite of food, we breathe in love with every breath, we think love with every thought, we express love with every word—because we know that not only is love the great healer, it is also the antidote for everything that creates arthritic conditions.*

So we must begin our quest for perfect joints by affirming our normal condition—health. We image ourselves as the perfect design we were created to mirror. We never think of ourselves or speak of ourselves as anything less than perfect. We don't identify ourselves with any limiting conditions by using such phrases as "*my* arthritis" or "*I am* an arthritic." We identify only with conditions of life. We speak words of life and joy and love—not only to ourselves, but to all around us. We examine our lives for conflict and, if we find any, we bless it and change it by bringing love into it. Love is the great emancipator. It elevates any conflict into the spiritual realm where it can no longer exist. *Love is patient and kind; love is not jealous or boastful; it is not arrogant or rude. Love does not insist on its own way; it is not irritable or resentful; it does not rejoice at wrong, but rejoices in the right. Love bears all things, believes all things, hopes all things, endures all things. (I Cor. 13:4-7)*

Laws of Body Renewal

So, love is the faculty we will use to elevate ourselves into the spiritual realm where we will become aware of our divine design. But on our journey, let us not forget about the laws that God designated to care for our bodies. Mary Katherine MacDougall says it well: *To help love along we take better care of our body than we ever have before. We eat the right food, we exercise, we rest. We thank our body for every bit of improvement and we constantly expect more. We expect healing.*

And we will get healing. We will be healed to the exact extent that we conform to all the laws of body renewal. We begin, of course, by seeking first the kingdom of God, and by aligning ourselves with the universal life force within us. Then, by obeying all of God's laws, we eventually will reach the point of perfection that we seek.

Putting Ourselves in Motion

Although this book does not deal specifically with exercise nor with specific exercises, the importance of regular body movement in any health-building program cannot be overlooked. It is essential. There is a tendency for many people manifesting arthritis to shun exercise because they are afraid of the pain involved. This is a valid concern but does not have to prevent at least *some* regular exercise. For example, arthritis manifesting in the fingers does not preclude a daily walk, nor does arthritis manifesting in the knees preclude a regular swim in a heated pool. The exercise does not necessarily have to be directed to the joint or joints in question. Regular exercise benefits the entire body, including all the joints. It increases the amount of oxygen in the blood, the circulation of the blood, and the opportunity for all of the cells to obtain the nutrients in the blood. It increases the ability of the bowels to remove waste matter and therefore toxins from our bodies. It helps alleviate stress (which some think to be one of the major causes of arthritis), and it makes us sleep better.

These are just a few of the many benefits of regular exercise. Choose an exercise appropriate for you. Consult your physician. He will help you decide which is best.

Protein Means Progress

As in any renewal, the renewal of the body involves a rebuilding of the body. And there is no rebuilding possible in the human body without good nutrition.

Good nutrition begins with good food, and good food begins with good protein. Proteins are the building blocks of life. With them God molds the tissues and sinews of His most precious creation. (See the special section for a list,

59

page 17.)

The importance of regularly ingesting top-grade protein cannot be overemphasized. An arthritis clinic in California instructs its patients to include at least two raw eggs in a glass of milk for breakfast and to drink an additional four to six glasses of certified raw milk and eat lots of cheese throughout the day! The directors of the clinic know that in order to rebuild tissue the body must have sufficient raw materials. Of course, this regime may not suit you, but it does point up the need for top-grade protein.

Choose Carbohydrates Carefully

The ingestion of "destructive" carbohydrates has much to do with exacerbating an arthritic condition. (Although they are not carbohydrates, coffee, alcoholic beverages, and spices of all kinds are also destructive to human tissues.)

The *constructive* carbohydrates containing the life force in abundance, as listed on page 20, are the ones from which we should choose.

Oil the Joints

No nutritional regime is complete without the addition of a good quality oil. We must not forget that we were designed as a frictionless miracle machine and, like all machines, we need oil. (See page 22)

In addition to a good raw salad oil like safflower oil, corn oil, sunflower oil, and many others that can be used on salads and vegetables, we should endeavor to ingest one or more teaspoonful of cod liver oil each day. Because of its good supply of vitamins A and D, cod liver oil has a special application in joint problems.

Cod liver oil has a distinctive taste so we will probably not want to use it on our food. It is available, however, in flavored forms as well as in capsule form. No matter which way you choose to take it, it is a good idea to use it.

Suggested Supplements

Recent research being done on the use of supplemental amounts of vitamins and minerals in arthritis cases is nothing short of spectacular. However, this research began at least twenty-five years ago when a Connecticut internist discovered a correlation between niacinamide (one of the B complex vitamins) and joint flexibility in his arthritic patients. More recently, studies done with this vitamin and with other B complex vitamins—riboflavin (B2), pyridoxine (B6), and pantothenic acid—show that the blood levels of these nutrients in arthritic people are significantly lower than that of non-arthritic people, in some cases by as much as seventy-five percent!

Scientists have noted that vitamin A is also in shorter supply in those suffering from arthritis, and they feel that they have reason to suspect the special importance of vitamin C and the minerals magnesium, calcium, manganese, phosphate, potassium, and copper!

Such a plethora of special nutrients! Is it possible to suspect that the body of one suffering from arthritis can be deficient in so many nutrients? The answer is that it is not only possible, it is highly probable!

We have already noted that joint problems can manifest when there is a deficiency of love in our lives. It is also possible to create problems for ourselves when there is an abundance of will and zeal and a deficiency of wisdom and understanding. God has bestowed on us all the aspects of His own nature in the form of twelve powers. We are an outpicturing of our attempt to harmonize these powers.

61

Although they are in infinite supply, our use of them can vary manifoldly. When we treat one or more of these powers as missing or in short supply, we will not have the "raw materials" we need in order to manifest our perfection. It is much the same in our own bodies. There are approximately forty nutrients needed by each of the one hundred trillion cells of our bodies. When one or more of these nutrients is missing or is in short supply, the cell will not have the raw materials it needs in order to manifest its perfect design.

The fact that such a battery of nutrients seems to be in short supply suggests the special importance of these nutrients in the health of the joint tissue. Certain tissues of the body, in addition to needing the normal amounts of many nutrients, have a need for additional amounts of certain others.

Years ago small boys used to get marched to the clothing store once a year to get an Easter outfit. This outfit included new shoes, socks, shirt, tie, and suit. Without any one of these items the outfit would not have been complete. Although all items were needed, some were more critical than others. Since small boys were never careful about how they treated their clothes, wise mothers would purchase suits with two pairs of trousers. All items were needed, but extra trousers were needed.

Such seems to be the case with joint cartilage. All the nutrients are needed, but certain nutrients seem to be needed in extra amounts. Each of the nutrients mentioned has a special biochemical application to the highly-specialized joint cartilage. For example, vitamins A and C and the mineral manganese are essential in the manufacture of the ground substance in the cartilage. Vitamin C is needed in the manufacture of collagen which makes up about sixty percent of cartilage.

Adrenal Glands Important

The adrenal glands are important because of their manufacture and release of cortisone-like hormones. These diminish inflammation and the destruction of the joint cartilage. The adrenal glands are induced to do this on command from the pituitary gland, which releases a hormone known as ACTH.

Riboflavin (vitamin B2) is involved in the release of ACTH from the pituitary. Vitamin C is needed in ACTH production for the adrenals. Also needed by the adrenals are vitamin A and the B complex vitamins niacinamide, pantothenic acid, folic acid, biotin, and pyridoxine (B6). These and other nutrients all have special application in the health of our joints. When they are insufficiently supplied in our diets, the cells of our joints cannot build according to the perfect plan.

It is important that we see to it that our diets are generously supplied with these nutrients. Eating the proper proteins, carbohydrates, and oils is a good place to begin. Good nutrition begins with good food. However, if we have reached the point where a condition such as arthritis has manifested, we probably need more help than food alone can offer. Dr. Roger J. Williams tells us that: . . . *on the basis of reports presently available, the items that certainly need to be considered are niacin, pantothenic acid, riboflavin, vitamin A, vitamin B6, vitamin C, magnesium, calcium, phosphate, and other minerals. The object is to feed* adequately *the cells that are involved in producing synovial fluid and in keeping the bones, joints, and muscles in healthy condition.*

Dr. Morton Biskind writing in "The American Journal of Digestive Diseases" states: *Tissues once depleted require much more of the essential factors than it is possible to ob-*

tain even in an optimal diet. It is, nevertheless, important that the diet be as rich in protein and vitamins as feasible. But the vitamin content of the diet may not be depended on *to yield quantities sufficient to heal nutritional [injuries]. Experience indicates that at least 10, 20, even 50 times the maintenance amounts for persons who have never been deficient are often necessary for therapy . . . .*

How much do we need? We will each have to decide for ourselves. It is always a good idea, however, to be sure that our nutritional program has a complete multiple vitamin-mineral formula as its basis. This might contain between 10,000 and 25,000 IUs of vitamin A, between 400 and 1,000 IUs of vitamin D, good amounts of vitamin E, some vitamin C, and about 10 or more milligrams of all eleven B complex vitamins. It should also contain all the major minerals and trace minerals. In addition to this we may consider extra amounts of vitamin C, B complex, and minerals.

The amounts of vitamin C suggested range from an RDA by the government of 60 milligrams per day to the suggestions of many scientists who say that, with a problem such as arthritis, between 3,000 and 15,000 milligrams daily would be more appropriate. Almost all researchers into the problems of arthritis realize the extreme importance of sufficient amounts of this vitamin. Let's be sure we are getting enough but begin with small amounts.

Because of the many B complex vitamins involved with joint health, it may be a good idea to take a very high-potency B complex (all eleven B vitamins) supplement *at least* once a day. Since the B vitamins work as a team, they should be taken as a team. If we feel we need more of one or two specific B complex vitamins, we can add these to our program.

A good multiple mineral tablet might round out our

program and ensure our supply of these important nutrients.

Two New Friends

In addition to these well-known nutrients, there are two supplements that have special significance in joint problems.

The first is a product made from the juice of the alfalfa plant. It is usually made into a supplement called alfalfa *juice* tablets (not to be confused with the tablets made only from the leaves and stems). This product has afforded many sufferers of arthritis relief from their pain when taken in sufficient quantity. Of course we each will have to decide what quantities are sufficient with each supplement.

The second product is the extract from a plant that has been used by the Indian tribes in this country and in Mexico for thousands of years.

Research done at two famous arthritis clinics has indicated that the regular use of the extract of yucca juice in tablet form may provide another weapon in the arsenal of nutrients available to the arthritis sufferer. Writing in "The Journal of Applied Nutrition," Drs. Robert Bingham and Bernard A. Bellew say: *The effectiveness of yucca saponin in relieving swelling, pain, and stiffness was evaluated . . . in both rheumatoid and osteoid forms of arthritis . . . (it) proved to have overall and specific beneficial effects. . . .* Patients took between two and eight tablets per day (average was four per day). The study indicated that yucca tablets are safe and very effective.

In a further study done by Drs. Bingham, Harris, and Laga, 212 arthritic patients . . . *were placed on high-protein diets with natural foods and were given exercise programs. . . . About two-thirds of all arthritic patients found some benefit from taking the yucca extract.*

Both yucca and alfalfa juice tablets are readily available in most health food stores or in special sections of super-markets.

First Things First

Well, there it is—a strategy for a return to health. The authors do not pretend that it is the only plan, but it is one that has worked for many people.

Of course the most important aspect of this program, the indispensable key to any renewal of our bodies, is the realization of our innate divinity. If we are to achieve the perfection for which we were designed, we must first accept the fact that we have a potential for that perfection. We must contact the life force within our bodies and allow it to fully express. We do this when we seek first the kingdom of God. In doing this, *all* else follows.

We don't improve our health merely by eating correctly and exercising. They are very important to be sure. But good food, regular exercise, and proper rest will take us only as far as the image that we have of ourselves, for we can never be more than we believe ourselves to be.

Let us image ourselves in the perfection that we are. Let us follow *all* God's laws of permanent body building, in-cluding optimum nutrition, regular exercise, and abundant fresh air and rest. And let us remember that before we do all these things, we must put God first in our lives. We can begin raising ourselves to the consciousness of God by prac-ticing the power of love on our neighbors and on ourselves.

When we can truly love the body and know that it is the temple of God—the dwelling-place of the Most High— we will immediately want to obey all the laws that protect and maintain that temple. When we love something, we always want to do the best for it. In this way, any dis-ease will disappear and we will be left with a physical body filled with the essence of purest love manifesting as perfect life.

So faith, hope, love abide, these three; but the greatest of these is love. (I Cor. 13:13)

Overcoming Overweight

When spiritual man (I AM) . . . makes use of the God ideas inherent in him, he brings forth the ideal body in its elemental perfection. These wonderful words of Charles Fillmore tell us very clearly that every human body instinctively seeks perfection. Each human body has a built-in blueprint that it was created to follow. This blueprint is always perfect. It is the real you!

That fact may surprise you if you are overweight. It shouldn't! Your body is right now seeking the slenderness and the perfection that are really you. The fact that it is not manifesting this slenderness indicates that there is something (or some things) inhibiting it from doing so.

If you are dissatisfied with your present shape—if it seems to be less than perfect—it is because you have not allowed the real you to come forth. You have somehow denied yourself. But, contrary to whatever sense of frustration or self-disapproval you might be experiencing, there really is a way to lose weight healthfully, enjoyably, and permanently. In fact, there is really only one way to do so—and that is to *gain your health,* because a healthy body will always result in the ideal weight. "But I am perfectly healthy," you say, "and I am still overweight!" The truth is that no one is perfectly healthy until he exactly mirrors his divine design; and no one exactly mirrors his divine design until he is perfectly healthy.

If we are interested in reclaiming our health, in seeking our divine birthright, then we must begin where all meaningful journeys begin—we must seek first the kingdom of

God. In seeking the kingdom of God, all that is rightfully ours will come to us. In seeking first the kingdom of God, all that we are meant to be will become manifest.

In the meantime, as we journey toward the kingdom of God, it is important that we realize that our present body form represents our present state of consciousness. We have been given the keys to the kingdom, it is true. But what we may not realize is that the keys can only be used to unlock our own minds.

Charles Fillmore once said: . . . *there is a definite relation between the thoughts of man and the conditions of his body.* It is impossible for us to be anything different from that which we believe ourselves to be. If we think of ourselves as "fat," then we will manifest fat in abundance.

It has been said that thoughts are things. Just as the body requires adequate physical nourishment in the form of food and drink, it also requires adequate mental nourishment from the thoughts we think. *Our bodies will always reflect our deepest beliefs about ourselves.* If we want to be slender and healthy, it is essential that we think of ourselves as slender and healthy.

Eight Steps Upward

There is a way of working with the divine intelligence within us. We have developed a program that has helped us and many others to get back in touch with their own bodies. We call it "Eight Steps Upward." It's as easy as ABC!

A is for *affirmations and denials.* In order to change our self-image, and ultimately our body image, there must be an assertion of that which is true about ourselves and a concomitant rejection of that which is false. And what is true? The truth (and we must affirm it) is that the divine cells of our bodies desire and seek only health and wholeness—

they seek only perfection. And we will become that perfection to the extent we allow it to express. And what is false? It is not true that overweight is a "normal" state, that some people are just "naturally fat." To believe this is to believe that the Creator would design something less than perfect. In order to impress these facts on our subconscious minds, we should repeat many times daily, either audibly or silently: *My divine body seeks slenderness and health.* And also, we can deny the inevitability of overweight by repeating: *Overweight is not my natural state.*

B is for *blessing.* We will only act in our own best interest when we love ourselves. And loving ourselves means loving the bodies God has given to us. What was our reaction to our bodies the last time we looked at ourselves in the mirror? Was it one of love and joy, or did we think thoughts of repugnance? Did we like what we saw? It is possible to love your body and not like the way it looks, just as there are times that we can love our children and not like the way they act. We must learn to discern between the two. We must look upon our bodies with love, for it is only when we love them that we will want the best for them. So let's bless our bodies. Let's bless the one hundred trillion cells that are working so relentlessly to express the perfection that we are. Each time we look in the mirror, let's say to our bodies: "I love you and I bless you as I strive to perfect you."

C is for *commitment.* The next step is to begin changing our consciousness with a firm commitment to slenderness and health. Unless we are strongly committed to improving ourselves, we run the risk of giving up before we have reached our goal. The faculty of zeal is essential or else we are like a powerful engine with no fuel. One of the most effective ways to show our commitment to slenderness and health is to write out what we want to accomplish in the form of a promise and sign it. We must make a covenant with our bodies.

D is for *deeds*. This is one of the keys to working with the divine intelligence within our bodies. *We must make an effort* on our own behalf. There is no other way! No one can fill our minds with uplifting thoughts for us; no one can eat good food for us; and no one can exercise our bodies for us. We can grow slimmer only by our own striving. Any desire must be followed by a deed if it is to manifest in our lives. To pray for weight loss and to desire slimness without wanting to expend an effort on our own behalf is to expect something for nothing. We can never work in opposition to the law of cause and effect—not even with prayer. In order for us to demonstrate the slimness we desire, we must perform a deed. A desire plus a deed will yield a demonstration. A desire without a deed is a dead end.

E is for *envisioning*. Among the most creative of the mind powers is our power to envision. We do this, of course, by using the imagination. There is no area where the powerful tool of imagination is more useful than in the area of weight loss. By consciously directing the imagination to hold a definite, firmly pictured goal, we will subconsciously direct our lives toward the attainment of that goal. What do we want to look like? How much do we want to weigh? These are questions we must ask ourselves. When we have decided on appropriate answers, we must create a firm image and hold that image in our minds. Every time we think of ourselves, it should be in this image. However, the image should be clear and definite. (Since most people do not begin getting overweight until after their twenties, a picture of ourselves at an earlier age will sometimes help the imagination get a clear image of what we want to look like. If overweight has always been a problem, cutting a picture of a slim, attractive person out of a magazine and pasting it in a conspicuous place can help to remind us of our goal.)

F is for *faith*. When we have committed ourselves to the first five steps, then we know that our faith will be anchored in the solid foundation of deeds. We can then have complete assurance that, having complied with God's laws, we will be compensated by God with the slimness and health we desire.

G is for *gratitude*. After placing our unshakable faith in the fact that God will answer our deeds, we should then give thanks. Our gratitude shows our faith and our trust in God.

H is for *hands off*. Once we have acted on our own behalf, placed our faith in and shown our gratitude to God, there is nothing more we can do. To do more would be to interfere with the universal life force unfolding within us. Therefore, we must keep our hands off and allow the perfect design to manifest.

The Calorie Connection

Before beginning the nutritional aspects of weight loss, it may be helpful to point out that one pound of body fat contains approximately 3,500 calories. Therefore, if we eat 500 calories less per day than we would normally eat, we will theoretically lose 1 pound per week (500 calories x 7 days = 3,500 calories or 1 pound).

Two pounds per week is generally the most that should be lost if the body is to remain healthy. Weight should never be forced off; it should be *coaxed* off. And let's not try to get by with any less than about 1,100 calories per day for women and about 1,500 calories per day for men. Less than this puts a dangerous strain on the body. Don't forget, we did not get overweight between Christmas and the New Year but between the New Year and Christmas.

A few more words about calories are probably in order. A calorie is actually a measure of heat. It is concerned with only one aspect of nutrition, and that is food energy. Obviously, the more energy a food yields the more movement it takes to "burn it up." What is not burned up is stored in the body in the various fat deposits.

While it is true that we must watch our calories, it is also true that we must *judge calories by the company they keep.* For example, a supper of six ounces of fish, two fresh vegetables, a salad, and a piece of fruit for dessert will yield the same number of calories as a four-ounce candy bar of chocolate-covered almonds. Which do you think is a better choice?

Now on to more specific information. Any body rebuilding or renewing requires proteins. Proteins, the correct ones in sufficient amounts, constitute an important key to vibrant health and proper weight. Next to water, protein is the most abundant substance in the body and, in fact, is needed if fluid balance is to be maintained. When there is too little protein, the tissues hold abnormal amounts of liquid and we become swollen and bloated.

It is a good idea when trying to lose weight to choose our proteins only from the top-grade ones. (See the special section, page 17, in the second chapter for vital information.)

Because of the high calorie-to-protein ratio of cheese, it should be used sparingly, if at all, during a weight-loss program. Cottage cheese, however, is still an excellent choice. Low fat is better than full-fat at this time. The same holds true for milk; skimmed milk is to be preferred over full-fat. Meats should be eaten lean and chicken and turkey unfried and skinless.

And how much protein should we eat? The number of grams of protein needed daily is determined by taking your *ideal* weight (*not* necessarily your present weight) and dividing by a factor of two. For example, if your present weight is 160 pounds but your target weight or *ideal* weight is 120 pounds, you should try to ingest about 60 grams of protein per day (120 pounds ÷ 2 = 60 grams of protein per day). Of course, this figure is only an approximation. You will have to determine how you feel when taking this amount. You may feel you need more or less.

Carbohydrates

The key word, especially in dealing with weight loss, is *constructive carbohydrates*. It is the non-constructive carbohydrates that cause most nutritional problems. The constructive carbohydrates are the complex, unrefined carbohydrates. They are: fresh fruit, fresh vegetables, whole grains, honey, blackstrap molasses, and pure maple syrup. (Although the last three are legitimate carbohydrates, because of their high caloric content it is wise to avoid them during weight loss.) Fruits, vegetables, and whole grains, in addition to being wonderful carbohydrates, have the added advantage of supplying the body with a good amount of indigestible bulk (or fiber). This bulk, in addition to filling the stomach, slows down the course of a meal and provides time for appetite satisfaction to supervene. Since this indigestible cellulose is not absorbed, it does not add to the body's caloric pool and therefore cannot add to the body's fat.

Notice that the list includes fresh fruit—not dried fruits and fruit juices. These are much too concentrated in sugar and should be avoided while trying to lose weight. (One could easily eat five or six prunes but would not consider eating five or six plums. Yet the same amount of sugar is in each!)

There are certain vegetables that should be eaten sparingly while losing weight. These are all of the vegetables which, because of their goitrogenic properties, can depress thyroid activity and slow the metabolism. The vegetables include the members of the brassica family—cabbage, broccoli, brussels sprouts, and cauliflower, as well as turnips, rutabagas, and soybeans.

Good vegetables to choose from are the squash family, green beans, salad greens, tomatoes, onions, artichokes, and carrots. Choose sparingly from the more starchy ones like potatoes, corn, and the like.

Grains generally have relatively more calories per serving than vegetables. Although they are an important part of a healthful diet, be careful not to overdo eating them.

When "Fat" Is Good

Good fats—the right kinds of fats—do not make excess fat in the body unless the entire diet is excessive. Fats in meals make them more satisfying, providing a higher satiety value since they are so slow to leave the stomach.

The most important nutritional value of fats for dieting purposes is the cells' need for linoleic acid—one of the essential fatty acids. The cells cannot make linoleic acid themselves; it must come from the foods we eat.

Good sources of linoleic acid are: safflower oil, corn oil, sunflower oil, and soy oil. These are the most desirable.

Eat these wonderful oils raw. They should not be heated, so they are not to be used for cooking. Use small amounts on salads, vegetables, toast, or any other way you can think to use them.

When losing weight the proper way, the body is being trained to establish a new metabolism. It is being rebuilt. In order to assure that all the nutrients are being introduced

75

into the body, it may be a good idea to supplement our diets with vitamins and minerals. Supplemental amounts of these important nutrients will ensure an adequate supply of vitamins and minerals so that all new tissue will be as perfect as possible.

Any good multiple vitamin-mineral formula should include adequate amounts of all the vitamins and minerals, including high amounts of all eleven of the B complex. This is our nutritional insurance.

Although the amount of "energy" we put into our bodies in the form of food must be monitored while reducing, the amount of "energy" we expend in the form of exercise is just as important.

Many obese persons are hesitant to engage in physical exercise because of the fear of increasing their appetites. However, many tests have shown this fear to be unfounded. Regular exercise is essential in any program of *permanent* weight reduction.

Dr. Jean Mayer, former head of the Department of Nutrition at Harvard University and an expert on obesity says: *Ideally, a person should exercise moderately (say, walk) for three-quarters of an hour or more every day and exercise vigorously on a bicycle ergometer or rowing machine for no less than fifteen minutes at least three times a week.* (It may be wise to consult your physician before vigorous exercise is attempted.)

To state it simply, exercise is the greatest device in keeping unwanted fat from returning.

Special Aids

To the extent that we succeed in changing our consciousness and implementing this change with the deeds that will rebuild and renew our bodies, to that extent we will

succeed in attaining the health and slimness we seek. However, just as we can use such techniques as affirmations and
denials and imaging to change our mental picture of ourselves, so too can we use special nutritional techniques to
change our physical image.

The liver is one of the key organs in any healthful and
permanent weight-loss program. The healthier the liver,
generally, the steadier and more permanent will be the
weight loss. Because of its unique ability to help detoxify
the liver by moving fat out of it, the B complex vitamin
choline has a very special significance. It is often combined
with the amino acid *methionine* (present in all top-grade
protein) and *betaine*. This combination of nutrients is called
a lipotropic formula. Often a lipotropic formula will also
contain the B complex vitamins *B12* and *inositol*. Whatever
the combination, it is a very helpful adjunct to any weight-
loss program. (Since the B complex vitamins work as a
team, be sure that your multiple vitamin-mineral formula
contains good amounts of all eleven of the B complex. This
will allow the lipotropic formula to work better.)

The ocean is rich in all the minerals needed in human
nutrition. Kelp, which grows in the sea and is actually a "sea
vegetable," is also rich in these nutrients. A good supply of
kelp helps to ensure us of at least a minimum supply of
many important minerals. However, its supply of trace
amounts of iodine is the important consideration in weight
reduction. Iodine is needed in tiny amounts by the thyroid.
The trace amounts of iodine in the kelp will help to supply
this important mineral so that the thyroid does not become
sluggish, thereby allowing the metabolism to become sluggish. A sluggish metabolism is not at all conducive to weight
loss and high energy output.

If you wish to use kelp in your program, take it after
breakfast and the noon meal. Some people find that if they

take kelp in the evening it keeps them awake at night. (Kelp does contain some sodium, so if you are sodium restricted, this aid is not for you at this time.)

Many Small Meals

It has been found that the eating of a single meal a day challenges the body to store more fat than if the same amount of food were ingested in a series of small meals. Therefore, when reducing, it is wise to plan your menu for the day and ingest the food in as many small meals as your life-style allows. A housewife who is at home all day obviously can plan many small meals more easily than someone who must work in an office all day. However, with a little imagination and preparation, it can be accomplished.

The authors have devised a blender drink that we call the Slimming Energizer. This drink can be made in the morning and sipped throughout the day in lieu of two meals. It is made as follows:

Mix in the blender the following (makes enough for two meals):

> 12 to 16 ounces of non-fat milk
> 1 or 2 raw eggs
> 1 tablespoonful of protein powder
>   (milk and egg type is best)
> ½ teaspoonful of safflower oil
> 1 tablespoonful of lecithin granules
> 1 tablespoonful of raw bran
> small piece of fresh fruit or 1 tea-
>   spoonful of honey (for taste)

We can use any fruit or combination of fruit and/or honey and/or vanilla flavoring to make the drink taste good. If it tastes good, we will be more prone to use it. (If for some reason you do not want to use milk, try using some watered-down papaya juice.)

This drink will yield about 550 to 600 calories (but what wonderful company these calories keep). However, since it will be used in place of two meals (usually breakfast and lunch), it yields not more than 300 calories per meal! It is a powerful drink, so we should sip it sl-o-o-o-w-l-y. It can be put in a thermos and taken to work and sipped on from time to time.

It is important to note the ingredients used and to know why they are used.

Milk is a top-grade protein food and a good source of many minerals, including calcium.

Eggs are the most perfect protein food and afford our bodies the finest building material. (If you are restricted from eating the yolks of eggs, use the whites only. However, realize that as you regain your health you will be able to include this wonderful food in its entirety in your diet.)

Protein powder is a concentrated food and will generally increase the amount of protein available without a proportional increase in the number of calories. Use a good-tasting one but not one containing sugar (sucrose). A milk and egg type protein powder is best. (Most of these are made with egg whites so that a yolk-restricted person can use them.)

Safflower oil is the most unsaturated of the vegetable oils and is highest in linoleic acid—essential to the cells.

Lecithin is high in the lipotropic vitamins and is also able to emulsify fat and cholesterol. In addition, it adds "smoothness" to the drink.

Since bran is a dietary fiber which is indigestible, it adds bulk to your meal without any calories. It can help to fill you up without filling you out! (If after using it for a few weeks you find that bran gives you too much gas, try taking less until the problem disappears.)

Fresh fruit or honey rounds out the drink, providing a wonderful constructive carbohydrate in addition to improving the taste.

This drink provides plenty of primary protein, good constructive carbohydrates, and an excellent oil. It is a high energy meal without being a fattening one. It can be used to begin a program of weight loss.

Supper during this time should consist of a medium serving of one of the primary proteins, a few good vegetables, a large salad, and a small piece of fresh fruit. A harmless beverage (like herb tea) would round it out. A supper such as this would not normally exceed about 600 calories. (If you get very hungry during the day, snack on a few celery sticks or carrot sticks or a few pieces of green pepper or cucumber. Keep some of these harmless snacks handy. If they are readily available, you will reach for them instead of reaching for something harmful and fattening. The more chewy it is, the more satisfying it will be.)

So between the Slimming Energizer (which we will consume for breakfast and lunch) and this supper, we will have ingested only about 1,100 to 1,200 calories, and each calorie is loaded with nutrition. We have made each calorie count and have presented our divine cells with the finest raw materials with which the life force within us can build the finest tissues.

Ultimate Success

Obesity can be overcome. It can be reversed. But it will take hard work and dedication. If obesity is to be "cured," the whole body must be "cured." The whole body must be brought into a better state of health.

It is important to remember that our bodies are chemical compounds. The thoughts we think, the foods we eat, and the exercises we perform affect that chemistry. If we conscientiously choose thoughts for their spiritual value, foods for their nutritive value, and exercises for their physiological value, our bodies will seek and ultimately attain the form and function that perfectly mirror their divine design.

Underweight Is Unnecessary

" . . . 'Man shall not live by bread alone, but by every word that proceeds from the mouth of God.' " (Matt. 4:4) It takes more than food to nourish a living human being.

There are many people who are proof of this statement. They eat what they consider to be a substantial amount of food each day and yet they remain underweight. Why?

To understand the situation, we first must realize that the mere act of putting food into the stomach does not, of itself, constitute nourishment. Eating does not mean we are actually fed. The truth of the matter is that we are only fed, or nourished, when the nutrients have actually gotten into the cells. Between the swallowing of food and its delivery to the cells, an entire world of chemical processes transpires. Persons who are underweight are undernourished. For some reason or other the nutrients are not getting into the cells where they can be utilized in building the body.

But we said there is more to nourishing a person than just food. The soul requires nourishment as much as the body does. Spiritual nourishment is craved by every soul if it is to grow. And just as with the body's nourishment, that of the soul must also be supplied regularly.

Underweight is an indication of lack of wholeness. It is physical health that is less than perfect. It means that the divine blueprint has not been totally followed. Thus it becomes a perfect opportunity to work with the God-given spiritual and physical laws that will lead us directly to that perfect design if we are willing to make the effort.

And what is this effort? It means putting God first in *all* things. This is a phrase we are apt to toss off lightly, agreeing with it intellectually but not taking it deeply into our hearts. God first! It has to be. The entire order of the universe is built on this principle.

If we separate ourselves from God, we lose communion with Him. This is not His fault; it is ours. God is still on the line, so to speak. It is we who have hung up the receiver!

The best way to make contact with God is through daily meditation. It is here that we obtain our spiritual sustenance. Meditation and prayer are the green pastures where our souls are restored and where we can spiritually feed. When we have this daily communion with the Creator of the universe, we begin to feel the flow of life as it permeates our bodies. We are strengthened, calmed, and nurtured by this life force within us.

During our times of meditation, we can envision the life force in the cells as it is at work turning essential nutrients into divine human tissue. We can direct our attention to the processes of digestion and assimilation, blessing these phenomenal functions and encouraging them to do their best.

The mind must be cleared of all negative elements that might be impeding the flow of nutrients to the cells. Search your consciousness over and over for traces of hindering thoughts and emotions. Dig them out and cast them away. You have no need of them. Make room for the good.

As the soul is able to fill more freely with the spirit of Christ, it experiences a sense of satiety. It feels nourished. This opens the way for the life force to better do its work of constructing the body temple. It becomes easier for the tissues to be strengthened and for new, healthy tissues to be clothed about the body. It is a movement toward wholeness.

The first step in gaining desirable weight, then, is gaining communion with God. Our goal is to have sound muscle tissue added to our frame, not fatty tissue. High-quality tissue is the objective. And high-quality soul development is where it all begins.

We must start to think of food in a new way. Rather than being entertainment and titillation to the taste buds, food must be regarded primarily as divine substance provided by the source of all substance for the regeneration and construction of the body temple. That is why blessing our food—saying grace—before we eat is a good idea. It helps to center our attention on the main purpose for eating: nourishing the life force within our cells.

Food regarded in such a manner—seen as divine appropriation for the physical body, which is none other than the expression of the Creator Himself—becomes a sacrament. Eating takes on religious or spiritual significance, as important as our prayers and affirmations. The life force within us becomes convinced of our desire to help it. It feels appreciated. These are all things we should think about in reference to eating.

Foods to Gain By

Then we come to the question of what to eat to help the body gain weight. There are definite guidelines for this—scientifically determined but nevertheless divinely ordained. As Myrtle Fillmore, cofounder of Unity, would remind us: *We must know the chemistry of the body; we must find the whole man. We have need of this outer man and we have to make the mortar that builds him up to a full development.*

Without sound principles by which to select our foods, eating becomes a hit-or-miss affair. If we are trying to gain some weight, we often try stuffing ourselves with "fattening" foods, merely to discover that the only gain might be a small bulge at the beltline. This is fat—not healthy muscle tissue. To gain solid tissue that enhances the body temple—both aesthetically and healthfully—we must learn the rules of good nutrition and make every effort to obey them.

Solid tissue is built of protein, so it is naturally to protein that we look first. We must remember that protein and *only* protein forms the basis for the weight improvement we are seeking. This is the kind of weight that will be distributed exactly where it should be and will be permanent.

Our protein foods are eggs, milk and milk products, cheeses (including cottage cheese), lean meat, fish, and poultry. These are the finest proteins, and each meal should be based on one of these life-building foods. Breakfast in particular must be scrutinized to make certain it is rich in protein.

(If you do not eat any foods from an animal source, you will have to scientifically combine your foods to provide the best amino acid balance. This is very tricky, so be careful.) The importance of the ingestion of top-grade protein cannot be stressed too strongly.

Each meal should also include a form of carbohydrate. Instead of the sugar, white flour, candy, cakes, alcoholic beverages, soft drinks, pastries, and the myriads of junk foods people ingest in their attempts to put on weight, eat some *constructive* carbohydrates that will provide the proper fuel for the body.

The life force requires one more type of food, and that is essential fatty acids. We know them as oils. One or two teaspoonsful or more daily of a good, cold-pressed, unpreserved oil can be beneficial. If you can use wheat germ oil as part of your daily quota, so much the better. (If you don't like the taste of wheat germ oil, it can be put into a blended

protein drink or taken in capsule form.) The popular vegetable oils, such as safflower, corn, sunflower, sesame, and
soy can be used on salads, baked potatoes and other vegetables, toast, and in soups and blender drinks. (And don't
forget Better Butter; see "Your Body's Nutritional Needs,"
page 24.) Remember to refrigerate these unpreserved oils
after opening them.

Three Secrets

One of the secrets of gaining healthful pounds is the
eating of at least three complete meals every day. Each
meal should contain at least protein and carbohydrates. It is
important not to skip a meal or skimp o meals. All of the
nutrients must be supplied if they are e⁄er to get into the
tissues.

Another secret of attaining more weight is the use of a
nourishing protein drink *in addition to* your regular meals.
This can be made in advance and carried with you to be
sipped *between* meals and even before bed, if you feel
hungry. There are many recipes for such a good-tasting,
nourishing drink. Here is a basic one you can alter to suit
your own taste. We call it the Body Builder.

Blend the following:

8 ounces of milk or juice
1 tablespoonful protein powder (milk and egg
    type is best)
1 raw egg
1 teaspoonful wheat germ oil (or any other
    good oil)
1 banana
1 teaspoonful of honey (or any of the other
    acceptable sweeteners)
1 tablespoonful of granular lecithin

This delicious drink will make one serving. Multiply the amounts to fit your eating pattern. There are numerous ways in which you can change the flavor of this drink. Peaches, strawberries, apples, or any other fruits can be substituted for the banana. Carob powder can be used as chocolate flavoring. A little experimentation will reveal the almost limitless taste nuances you can devise. Since the drink should be used every day, it will always be appealing to you because its flavor (and texture) can be changed whenever you wish.

Another suggestion for between-meal "meals" is raw, unsalted nuts and seeds. They not only are excellent sources of trace minerals but they are also rich in essential oils. They are good tasting, too!

The third nutritional secret of gaining weight is the use of digestive enzymes. Often we do not derive the maximum nutritive value from our foods because we are not breaking them down properly. Our bodies may lack adequate amounts of digestive enzymes. We are eating the right foods in the right amounts but they are not doing us the good they should. In other words, the freighter was loaded but somehow the goods never reached port—the food was eaten but the nutrients never reached the cells. And we must keep in mind that we are not really nourished until the cells receive the raw materials required for sustaining and building life.

Digestive enzymes, taken as a supplement after each meal, can help our body temples to get the most benefit out of our food. Taking a multiple enzyme tablet containing pancreatic and other enzymes can therefore be a wise practice. (If you have a stomach ulcer it may be wise to consult your physician before choosing an enzyme.)

Total Nutrition

In addition to the three nutritional secrets to healthful weight gain, there are some basic supplements we should consider. Are you taking a high-potency, multiple vitamin formula? Are you taking, in addition, a complete B complex that contains all eleven of the B vitamins? Are you getting enough vitamin C? (Many researchers are advising 1,000 to 5,000 milligrams daily). What about minerals? Extra calcium or a multiple mineral complex is always helpful.

The life force really needs *all* of the nutrients—all of the vitamins and minerals—to create more life within us. There are certain things it does *not* want, however, and we should avoid these cell-assassins as if our lives depended upon it. (They do!)

Things like caffeine, narcotics, tobacco, and alcohol do not belong in the body temple. These substances tear us down, destroying nutrients and weakening the life of our cells. They inhibit the building of solid muscle tissue and tend to hold the weight below its natural level.

Meditation can be used to help overcome these villains. See and regard yourself as a *non*-smoker or *non*-drinker. Make contact with your Christ self, be in awe of the power it possesses, and lovingly try to provide that Christ Spirit with the best home you can give it. We come into obedience to God's physical laws through obedience to His spiritual laws. Myrtle Fillmore was always aware of the need for obedience to the laws of both realms, the spiritual and the physical: *There is also a physical side to the operation of this divine law. The body and its needs must have our consideration. We must not drive the body or neglect its normal needs.*

Mrs. Fillmore has introduced another important aspect here. If we want to gain weight (and thereby gain health), we must not push the body too much. We need to get the proper rest and sleep during each twenty-four-hour period. This gives the body a chance to "catch up." It gives the nerves a rest and helps to keep us from burning up nutrients unnecessarily. Develop regular and adequate sleep patterns along with several "rest breaks" whenever possible during the day if you want your body to function at its best.

This doesn't mean that we should not exercise, however. Proper sleep and rest are health "musts," but so is regular physical exercise. The proper exercise can improve circulation, the means by which the nutrients are delivered to the individual cells. It also tends to have a calming, stabilizing effect upon the body, which is certainly to be desired. In addition, exercise keeps the muscles toned and firm, after their true design.

We must not ignore physical exercise. Choose the type with which you are most comfortable and do it regularly. Walking, cycling, swimming, yoga—these are all excellent examples. Whatever type you select must be done enthusiastically but not to the point of exhaustion. Do add exercise to your weight-gaining regime. It is a great body equalizer.

It might be wise to point out that some people who consider themselves to be underweight are not underweight at all. A slender body is healthier than a plump one. The astounding thing about the body is this: Once good health is attained, your "normal" weight is automatically attained as well.

If you are among those who feel the need to improve their health and thus increase their weight, trying to achieve this may not have been easy for you up to now. But with the suggestions presented here, you might discover the answer. We can always count on the wisdom of the life force to help regenerate our bodies once we have done our share. If we have begun to change our consciousness, lifting it to attunement with the perfect blueprint of our Christ selves, and if we have begun practicing the principles of good nutrition and exercise, we can expect to attain the proper weight. The life force is aware of what that proper weight is and will bring us to it if we will give it the opportunity to do so.

Let us concentrate on providing the divine sculptor with the finest materials. When we do so, we can rest assured that He will fashion a body so fine that every cell of it will sing His praises.

Insomniacs, Awaken to Wholeness

If you sit down, you will not be afraid; when you lie down, your sleep will be sweet. (Proverbs 3:24)

Sleep—that mysteriously suspended state the physical body seems to require on a regular basis—is a blessing easily taken for granted by those to whom it comes freely. But for the millions of people who do not enjoy sound, restful sleep, life can be an agonizing experience. And that should never be, for life should (and can) be a joyful experience.

Perhaps you might want to look at sleep in a new way. By changing aspects of your consciousness and thought patterns, along with changing your dietary and exercise patterns, you will discover how readily you can have a *little sleep, a little slumber* . . . as mentioned in Proverbs 24:33.

Physically, the body seems to require sleep in order to efficiently repair and regenerate the cells, particularly the nerves. There have been numerous scientific studies done on the phenomenon of sleep, yet there are still many aspects of it that remain a mystery. But this need not bother us. What we need to know is that it is necessary at this stage of our unfoldment to receive rest and sleep on a regular basis and that this sleep can be successfully attained by making a few modifications in our lives.

Sleeplessness interferes with the natural rhythm of the body. And, because we are a part of a universe whose very design is one of order and rhythm, we must establish good rhythms in our own lives. All life reflects an ebb and a flow—periods of activity and periods of rest. Did not even the great Creator rest on the seventh day? And did not Jesus admonish His disciples to restore and refresh themselves: *And he said to them, "Come away by yourselves to a lonely place, and rest a while."* (Mark 6:31)

Charles Fillmore discusses the importance of sleep in *Atom-Smashing Power of Mind: During sleep the system, under natural law, seeks to equalize the vital forces, and it does so if the intellectual concentration has not been too great.*

Sleep is an activity that consumes between one-quarter and one-third of our lives. It is safe to assume that it is crucial to our physical well-being.

There is another reason that sleep is so important to us, especially if we are students of metaphysics. Mr. Fillmore describes this most important reason in *Jesus Christ Heals: When we are in peaceful sleep, the outer clamor of thought is stilled and the great Spirit of the universe communicates its higher vision to the inner consciousness of man.* In other words, it is during sleep that we can receive divine ideas, wisdom, and inspiration that perhaps are not able to flow through into our subconscious minds when we are awake and involved in the bustle of our daily activities.

This valuable aspect of sleep was known even by the ancients. In Job 33:15-16 we read: *"In a dream, in a vision of the night, when deep sleep falls upon men, while they slumber on their beds, then he opens the ears of men, and terrifies them with warnings."*

There is no doubt that God can speak to us only when we are silent enough to hear Him. *Silence. It is the "pearl of great price," the spiritual balancer of all that is. At night you are blessed by it as you sleep,* writes Clara Palmer in *You Can Be Healed.* What better reason could there be for desiring good sleep than that of its serving as a time of our receptivity to the Father's voice?

We all know that any problem manifesting in our lives is, in essence, spiritual in nature. That is, we have "forgotten who we are." We have eschewed our oneness with our Creator. It is important to keep this in mind so that we don't fall into the trap of believing that, if we change a few things in our lives, like eating and exercising, we will manifest perfect health. These changes *alone* can never bring us perfection unless we *first* seek the kingdom of God. In other words, when we put God first, all else will follow. With this admonition firmly attached in our minds, let us now try to determine why it is that so many people are troubled by sleeplessness. What causes it? We in the Truth movement know that for every effect there is a cause.

Basically, insomnia is the result of anomalies or irregularities in the physical and/or the mental areas of our lives. By mental anomalies we mean, for example, the inability to relinquish worry, anxiety, fear, or plans for the future. By physical anomalies we mean any number of bodily discomforts, such as ambient heat or cold, lumpy mattress, bodily aches and pains, or other physical conditions that keep the attention focused on the body.

Let us look first at the mental factor—that of worry and fear. There are numerous passages in the Bible that address the subjects of fear and anxiety. (Apparently this has been a long-time weakness of humanity.) In John 14:27 Jesus said: ". . . *Let not your hearts be troubled, neither let them be afraid.*" And in Exodus 33:14 the Lord tells Moses: . . . *"My presence will go with you, and I will give you rest."*

In reality there is nothing at all to fear when we put our attention on God. Then there can only be that deep sense of peace of which the Psalmist spoke: *In peace I will both lie down and sleep; for thou alone, O Lord, makest me dwell in safety.* (Psalms 4:8)

We can all appreciate those words, can't we? But where do we begin in our attempt to relinquish worries and slip into peaceful slumber? Let's get practical and see what we can do.

There seems to be little doubt that relaxation of the body, followed by relaxation of the mind, is the first step in overcoming worry, fear, and restlessness. So, let's begin by breathing slowly and deeply, calling on divine love to help.

Relax. Mentally talk to each part of the body, starting from the feet up, telling it to relax and release. When you have succeeded in relaxing the entire body, take a deep breath and focus attention on the heart area. Continue to breathe deeply and meditate on words and ideas of love.

Call on Love

Catherine Ponder, in "The Healing Secret of the Ages," reminds us: . . . *words of love have a balancing effect upon the mind and body.* She further elaborates on the love power: *Love is a mind power native to man and exists in every one of us. It may be called forth and developed to bring about harmony among those who have been disunited through misunderstanding, contention, or selfishness.*

Loving feelings are necessary, therefore, in the attainment of the harmony and peace required for sound sleep. All conflicts are to be resolved and all negative feelings washed away in a flood of loving joy. Further ideas on this can be found in Charles Fillmore's pamphlet entitled *A Sure Remedy,* from which these words are taken: *See all things and all persons as they really are—pure Spirit—and send them your strongest thoughts of love. Do not go to bed any night feeling that you have an enemy in the world. Love* and forgiveness—good instruments of peaceful sleep. Perhaps the old saying that a guilty conscience keeps us from sleep is based on Truth after all! At any rate, it might be a good idea to check it out for yourself. If there is any need for forgiveness, do so at once, releasing everything and everyone to the highest good. Soon you will feel a pleasant sense of peace and relaxation flow through your body, all tensions and worries clearing away so that the blessing of sleep may come upon you.

Don't Be Concerned

At this point it is helpful to release all concern about not sleeping, because where there is concern there cannot be relaxation. We need to put ourselves into the Father's hands each night as we relax our bodies onto the bed. *Cast your burden on the Lord, and He will sustain you . . . .* (Psalms 55:22)

The Unity pamphlet *Health Through Spiritual Methods* introduces yet another idea. Good sleep is something that results from not only our bedtime thoughts but from those of the daytime as well: *As you steadily let thoughts of God and Truth occupy your mind and accompany you in all that you do throughout that day, there will be no question about your night's rest. You will grow to trust God perfectly. The secret of restful, strengthening relaxation is trust. This trustful relaxation is the remedy for sleeplessness as well as for many other ills.*

As the trusting sheep look to the shepherd, we can look with total trust to our God and know that . . . *he makes me lie down in green pastures. He leads me beside still waters; he restores my soul.* (Psalms 23:2, 3)

Use It for Good

Now here is something you may not have thought of as you lay there tossing and fretting: Those wakeful moments can be utilized productively! Hear what Ernest Wilson has to say in his pamphlet *He Giveth His Beloved Sleep: Make your waking state a time of meditation upon Truth. Memorize and repeat some of the affirmations and prayers that especially appeal to you.* An excellent idea.

While we are waiting for sleep, we have a wonderful opportunity to enjoy the luxury of unhurried thought, which is something a busy day does not afford us. We should take advantage of this delicious tidbit of time, allowing ideas to come through to us and then leisurely examining them. We will find that we will stop resenting these periods of wakefulness and, eventually, sleep will come.

One word about fear before we move on to the physical aspects of sleeplessness and some nutrition suggestions. If you need extra help in dealing with fear and anxiety, we suggest you read May Rowland's pamphlet entitled *What Are You Afraid Of?* She explains how *most fears take to their heels if we do something about them.* And we each do have it in our power to do something about them. We *can* control our thoughts and focus on God, the good.

Remembering our original premise in the first chapter of this book that Spirit, soul, and body are inextricably bound, let's take a look at what physical contributions we can make to overcome sleeplessness.

Very often, due to a combination of mental habits and nutrition deficiencies, our bodies get bogged down in a rut. We repeat these patterns over and over again, deepening the rut with each repetition. In the case of insomnia, the more we let it go on, the more it grows into a permanent pattern.

What is needed then is a determined effort to break the pattern. The body, which loves the security of a habit, can be taught to move into another "groove" and establish a new pattern—in this case, that of sound sleep. This retaining is accomplished through proper spiritual and mental orientation, as already discussed, along with proper diet and exercise.

Eat Better to Sleep Better

Nutrition plays a large role in strengthening the nerves and relaxing the daily tensions in our body temples. We must not forget the needs of the temple, for when they are not met, there is unrest expressed in some form or other. Proper nutrition, therefore, is worth investigating.

Proper nutrition, of course, begins with good food, and good food begins with adequate protein, constructive carbohydrates, oils, vitamin/mineral supplements, as mentioned in pages 17 through 34.

Some specific notes regarding nutrition and sleep:

The amino acids found in protein are necessary for proper sleep. In fact, one of the amino acids is sold separately as an aid to sleep: l-tryptophan. But if we eat adequate amounts of protein we will be getting our tryptophan.

Studies have shown that eating refined sugar and junk food health-wreckers is often the cause of disturbed sleep. Often that wakeful state is due to the ingestion of these delicious but malicious substances. They do not belong and will inevitably come back to haunt us in some manifestation or other along the way. Perhaps they can be compared to the money-changers whom Jesus threw out of the temple! There are certain things that simply do not belong.

We must be sure to get adequate amounts of oil in our

diets. This is important. It keeps us running smoothly. Dietary oils are also present in raw nuts and seeds, which are very good sources.

What about vitamins? Are we getting enough complete B complex? (There are eleven B vitamins in the complete complex.) This can help the nerves. But we must be sure not to take it in the evening if we have trouble sleeping, because it could then have the reverse effect and keep us awake. This advice goes for vitamin C as well, and for the mineral supplement kelp, which can stimulate the brain too much to allow it to relax and drift into sleep. It is best, therefore, to take the B complex, vitamin C, and kelp with the morning and noon meals only.

Minerals can do much to help us relax. They soothe the nerves and relax the muscles. Extra calcium and magnesium have been found by many to be especially helpful. They can be taken during the day and before bedtime. A good trick is to lightly chew or crush some calcium/magnesium tablets and take them with warm water or warm milk at bedtime. This can be very soothing and, in fact, can be repeated during the night if necessary.

Many people have weaned themselves from "sleeping pills" and other drugs by inching their way off the drugs and onto the calcium and magnesium. It only makes sense because, after all, calcium and magnesium are integral components of the human body whereas narcotics and drugs certainly are not!

Move More to Sleep More

In Ecclesiastes 5:12 it says: *Sweet is the sleep of a laborer* . . . We all have had the experience of a good night's sleep after a hard day's work. This indicates that adequate physical exercise results in better and more complete relaxation. How are we doing in this area? We might try some good regular exercise. Nothing beats a brisk walk. It is the least that we should do. If other types of body exercise (such as bicycling, jogging, swimming, jumping rope, yoga, etc.) appeal to you, do them. The life force within us is an active, moving thing and wants—no *needs*—to be used.

And here is a bonus we can derive from exercise. Dr. Henry C. Link, author of "The Return to Religion," claims that most fears are due to *an overactive mind and an underactive body.* Exercise, then, helps us in the mental areas as well as the physical. This should really be no surprise when we realize that the brain is part of the body. It responds to the same laws of physics and chemistry to which the rest of the body temple responds.

Keep in mind that the answer to any search for wholeness lies in the threefold nature of man: Spirit, soul, and body. We have discussed metaphysical ideas for you to consider and work with, as well as nutrition and exercise suggestions. We need to do it all. Partial efforts give partial success.

Total effort can only result in total success. That's the law! In which case it won't be long before you are able to tuck your body temple into bed, relax, think such reassuring words as: *Be still and know that I am God,* and very soon—z-z-z-z.

Don't Settle For Senility

Perched atop a bundle of nerves averaging not quite a yard long sits one of the most remarkable creations in the entire universe. This small, pink-gray mass of rubbery, moist cells never rests. It registers sounds, images, smells, tastes, pain, and pleasure. It regulates hormone production, heartbeat, metabolism, digestion, and elimination. It receives, analyzes, interprets, and transmits millions of signals each second, coordinating the movement of more than 600 muscles. It is a storehouse of past, present, and future information. It envisions dreams and harbors hopes. But as awe-inspiring and miraculous as these deeds appear, they cannot compare to this one unique attribute: It is the only structure in the universe capable of contemplating its own Creator! We are referring, of course, to that diminutive marvel of creation, the human brain.

Not only is the wonderful brain capable of contemplating its Creator, its very existence is essential if we are to communicate *with* our Creator. It is only when we have a brain that we can express ourselves. Charles Fillmore said it best: *When a man relinquishes his hold on brain and nervous system, he gives up the only avenue through which he can adequately express himself.* Without a brain, we can neither be impressed with the grandeur of creation nor can we express as a part of that grandeur.

In short, without our brains, we are simply incoherent masses of chemicals, incapable of expressing life. Things which inhibit the full potential of the brain, therefore, inhibit a full expression of life. Senility is just such a life-inhibitor and must be overcome if the body is to express its perfection.

Senility is one of those phenomena which seem to defy definition. Like courtesy, no one can define it properly but everyone recognizes it when he sees it. Medical texts define senility as . . . *pertaining to or characteristic of old age.* Since we in Truth don't believe that time is toxic or that time by itself can cause anything, it might be more appropriate to define senility as an outward manifestation of malnutrition of the brain.

The brain can starve nutritionally, but it can also starve spiritually. We know that the first step we always must take in regaining health is one of spiritual alignment; we must seek the kingdom of God—come in contact with our true Christ nature.

In the case of senility, however, it is not always possible to do this if the condition is advanced. We cannot expect a childlike mind to sit and meditate on abstract ideas. Or can we? Cannot even a child begin to understand the fundamental Truth of his own being when it is presented to him in loving, simple terms? The point is, however, that someone *else* may have to take over the job of meditating and imaging if the brain seems incapable of doing that itself at this time.

Thus, we as loving friends or relatives will begin to image the person as perfect and in full command of all of his faculties, despite any appearances to the contrary. We must hold a steady picture—never wavering—of the perfection and vibrancy which are the rightful state of the person.

If, on the other hand, *you* are the one facing the challenge and you have reason to feel that your brain function is not what it should be, you can begin this very day to restore your brain to its former function—and beyond!

You will image yourself as youthful in appearance and

brain function—quick of step and quick of mind. Be very conscientious about setting time aside each day for quiet meditation in which you make contact with the life force, nourishing it with your thoughts and feelings of praise for the youthful activity it expresses in your mind and body.

Use your thinking power and your speaking power to decree words of Truth to your brain—the Truth being that there is no limit to its potential once we open ourselves to the flow of the life force. Charles Fillmore said: *We can praise our abilities, and our very brain cells will expand and increase in capacity and intelligence when we speak words of encouragement and appreciation to them.*

Living in the Now

Do not let your thoughts dwell in the past, for this is stagnation. Life is a forward movement; and if we want life, we must progress with it. Live in the now with your energies focused on the day at hand. In reality, there is *only* the now. That is all we ever have.

Jesus was adamant in His caution that we: *Take . . . no thought for the morrow: for the morrow shall take thought for the things of itself.* (Matt. 6:34 A.V.) Dwelling in the future is just as unsound as dwelling in the past. It is fine (and necessary) to have goals and plans for the future, but to live for them to the exclusion of the present is folly. *Nothing* is as important as the present time—that is where the work of our soul development is done. If we live counting the days until the arrival of some future event, that event arrives and passes and we have lost the precious golden moments of the *now* all along the way.

Our lives then become like the lines of this poem from an unknown author:

> *Spring is past,*
> *Summer is gone,*
> *Winter is here,*
> *And my song that I was meant to sing*
> *Is still unsung.*
> *I have spent my days*
> *Stringing and restringing my instrument.*

Let us take full advantage of each moment as it comes to us. Each is a precious gift from the Almighty, given to us to use in our search for the kingdom of God. We must remember always that the kingdom of God is at hand. It is here—now—if we will but attune ourselves to it. Let us play the song of life now and stop restringing our instruments.

Exercise is always an integral part of any health-building program. Physical exercise increases the circulation and brings rich oxygen-carrying blood to the entire body, including the brain.

Brisk, long walks (you may want to begin with short ones) are excellent for invigorating the tissues of the brain. Yoga has helped many. And fifteen minutes a day on a slantboard may be extremely beneficial. If you are going to use a slantboard, be sure to *begin with only a minute or two a day* and work up very gradually at your own pace to ten or fifteen minutes. Also—and this is very important—rise up from the slantboard *very, very* slowly and easily, otherwise too much blood may leave the head too quickly. This is extremely important. But do remember to exercise regularly. We need to move if we are to improve.

Exercising the Brain

Exercising our muscles is not enough. We must also take care to exercise the cells of our brains. This can be done not by engaging the brain cells in calisthenics but by challenging the brain and by memorizing!

The more we memorize, the better our memory and recall will become. This will be true not only with regard to the material recently memorized, but for material committed to memory long ago.

What should we memorize? How about some Shakespeare? Perhaps some Truth affirmations. Maybe a favorite chapter from the Scriptures, or a poem. It really doesn't matter as far as the brain is concerned. Just memorize. (The memorizing of Truth affirmations does have other benefits, however. It helps impress the subconscious mind with the Truth. This in itself brings great benefits.)

Experiments done with groups of laboratory animals have shown that when these animals were segregated and one group was given challenging games to play, their brains grew heavier, thicker, and richer than the other group which did not have these challenges.

Chess is a challenging game, as is bridge. Even checkers can be challenging to some. Solving crossword puzzles or mathematical problems is fun and food for the brain. Why not try to solve simple arithmetic problems in your head instead of using a calculator? Anything that challenges the brain exercises it. And the brain does need exercise if it is to retain its function.

Don't "Pass the Time"

It has been determined that those who are alert and sharp-witted all their lives are generally those who have a real interest—a purpose—in their lives. Too often when people retire they slip into a world of boredom and petty activitives with which they "pass the time." How dreadful! Life should always be stimulating and inspiring. It should have *meaningful* activity—activity that serves to strengthen our own souls and physical bodies as well as activity that shares our light with others, for we *are* our brother—we are all one.

Retirement can be a unique opportunity for our own growth. More time can be devoted to life and the life force within us. There is not space in this chapter to expand on this, so we strongly recommend a book overflowing with life-giving, anti-age ideas: Russell Kemp's *Live Youthfully Now,* a Unity publication. It suggests wonderful and realistic ways in which we can overcome our race ideas about age and all negative beliefs regarding it.

As we can see, the brain is an organic part of the body that must follow the physical laws if it is to maintain its proper functioning. Too often we see signs of approaching senility and resignedly attribute it to "old age," not realizing that there are definite reasons that this is happening. That is why Myrtle Fillmore made this remark: *Those who do not understand begin to say, "He is getting old." Not so; he's simply disobeying the health rules!* And she was absolutely right.

We have already seen the importance of the rules of exercise. Let us turn now to the rules of nutrition.

As we have mentioned before, our bodies are chemical compounds composed of billions of tiny cells. Each cell is an individual entity working laboriously at its one task—bringing us life. Each tiny cell is a chemical factory designed by an omniscient Creator solely for this purpose. We will have attained perfect health only when each cell of our bodies perfectly mirrors its divine design. If one part of the body is not functioning according to its divine design, it means that the entire body is out of balance. We must correct the chemistry of the whole body and then all parts will function properly as the entire body sings with the harmony of success.

Since all life takes place on the cellular level, we are not nourished until the nutrients actually get into the cells. It is as simple as that. Let's not forget that the brain is part of the body and that the *only* way brain cells can get their nutrients is from the circulating blood. When brain cells do not get sufficient nutrients they die and, once dead, the cells of the brain are not replaced! If anything interferes with the delivery of the nutrients in the blood to the waiting cells, the cells cannot perform as they were designed to do. When enough brain cells are thus affected, the actions of the brain will be discordant; therefore, the actions of the person will be discordant, and we will judge his behavior as being aberrant.

Our object, then, should be to keep these brain cells as healthy as possible. The only way to do this is to give them exactly what they need in the way of nutrients. However, let's remember these important facts:

1) The brain is part of the body, and all mental problems are ultimately physical problems.

2) The brain cells can obtain only those nutrients from our blood that we have provided through the foods we eat.

Dr. Harold Rosenberg, former President of the International Academy of Preventive Medicine, in his "Book of Vitamin Therapy" states: . . . *senility itself may be just a form of chronic malnutrition.*

The brain is part of the body and responds to the same laws of nutrition to which the rest of the body does. The body needs about forty nutrients every day. If it gets these nutrients, the entire body (including the brain) will be satisfied. As Myrtle Fillmore once said: . . . *we need to make practical all the knowledge we have concerning bodily renewal, through using intelligence and discrimination in the selection of our food.*

And science is learning every day what we need. Dr.

John Moriarty, MD writes in the "Journal of Applied Nutrition": . . . *optimum nutrition is highly important in the prevention and treatment of . . . mental disorders. A basic dietary regime includes: 1) a high protein intake derived from meat, fish, poultry, milk, eggs, and cheese; 2) a moderate total fat intake but plentiful in essential fatty acids (unsaturated oils); 3) a minimum or near zero ingestion of refined carbohydrates such as sucrose and white flour, with carbohydrates being derived chiefly from fruits and vegetables; 4) appropriate multivitamin supplementation.*

There can be no rebuilding or renewing without protein. It is the "bricks and mortar" with which God fashions our tissues. It is essential that we eat sufficient amounts of top-grade proteins at each meal. And the top-grade proteins are exactly the ones that Dr. Moriarty has listed. They are (in order of highest biological activity): eggs, milk and milk products, cheese, and flesh foods (fish, fowl, and lean meats). These are the finest building materials available. We do not have to eat *all* these super foods, but we should choose our protein from this list.

Maintenance, growth, rebuilding, and renewing depend on proteins. Let's treat our bodies to the best.

The area of nutrition where most Americans make their biggest mistake is in carbohydrates. It is the ingestion of the "destructive" carbohydrates that can cause so much trouble in the brain and body. These destructive carbohydrates are foods from which the life force has been denuded by the refining process. According to John Loughran in his classic book "The Bionomy of Power," *You can weaken your brain by persistently eating debased, denatured and refined foods. You can strengthen your brain . . . by good foods . . . containing all, not merely some, of the elements.*

Please refer to chapter two (pages 20 to 34) for a list of

constructive carbohydrates, proper oils, and vitamin/mineral supplements.

You can also use Better Butter on toast. Try not to forget to obtain your important oil every day.

As has already been mentioned, we are made up of a community of billions upon billions of tiny, hardworking cells. These cells are joined together to form the most marvelous "machine" in the universe—the human body. In order to make this machine run, the cells need fuel; and a very specific kind of fuel is best. That fuel is glucose. The more efficiently this glucose is distributed to the cells, the smoother the operation of the body.

All the cells of the body can burn glucose. Most of the cells can, in an emergency, utilize fat. The glaring exceptions to this are the cells of the brain and central nervous system. *When the brain doesn't get enough glucose it cannot function properly.* This deprivation can manifest as fatigue, depression, loss of memory, and other mental aberrations including senility. The brain needs fuel. Without fuel it cannot function correctly. Therefore, any interference with the step-by-step breakdown of glucose for the brain will result in impaired mental functions.

With these facts in mind, let's take a look at some special considerations.

B Complex

The B complex vitamins are essential in converting food into glucose and are also essential for the health of the nerves. Although certain members of the B complex family seem to be more concerned with mental health than others, they all work as a team and are all needed if health is to be attained and sustained. It may be a good idea to supplement the diet with one or two high-potency B complex tablets each day. (Be sure your tablet contains all eleven of the B complex.)

There is evidence that the B complex vitamins B1, B2, and niacin are in short supply in people manifesting senility. And at least one investigator has concluded that the addition of B6 to an otherwise healthy diet may reverse a loss of motivation and memory.

In their classic reference text "Modern Nutrition in Health and Disease," Drs. Goodhart and Shils write: *According to one group of investigators, B-complex vitamins and ascorbic acid [vitamin C] supplements have resulted in improved "general vitality and vigor" among the aged studied. According to others, administration of . . . [these vitamins] . . . has resulted in improvement in symptoms previously attributed to . . . senility. . . ."*

Vitamins C and E

The role of vitamin C in the body is so all-encompassing that even a slight deficiency puts a great strain on the body. It has been successfully used as part of a broad nutritional program in treating all types of mental problems. There is no doubt that it is essential if the brain cells are to receive optimum nutrition.

Add to this its use as an antioxidant which (along with vitamin E) slows down the "aging" process and we can see that vitamin C is an integral part of any program to restore the body to its original plan of perfection.

The internationally renowned surgeon Dr. Alton Ochsner believes: *There is . . . evidence that vitamin C administration is of value in preventing clotting within the veins.*

Many investigators suggest taking between 1,000 and 5,000 milligrams of vitamin C each day. Others suggest as much as 10,000 milligrams daily. We will each have to decide on our own optimum intake.

Since the delivery of glucose to the waiting cells of the brain is essential to the health of the brain, anything that interferes with that delivery is harmful. We must be sure that our arteries, veins, and small capillaries are kept open so that the delivery is effortless and complete.

There is much evidence to suggest that vitamin E, as well as vitamin C, prevents the unnatural clotting of blood and will assist the free flow of nutrients to the waiting cells.

One of the world's leading authorities on vitamin E, Dr. Wilfred E. Shute, M.D. states: *There can be no question about the superb antithrombin, [anticlotting] activity of alpha tocopherol [vitamin E]. . . .*

Glutamic Acid

We know that, without fuel, the brain cells cannot function at all and that the main fuel for the brain is glucose. There is something else, however, that brain cells can and do use for fuel. It is an amino acid—one of the building blocks of protein—called glutamic acid. Glutamic acid is the only amino acid that can be metabolized by the brain. It has not been found to be essential as far as the rest of the body is concerned. However, it can be and is readily used by the brain for fuel. It is *uniquely* a brain fuel and as such must be a special consideration when dealing with any mental aberrations such as senility.

Since glutamic acid is an amino acid, it is present in all the top-grade protein foods. It is also available in supplemental tablet and powder form. The powdered form can be blended into drinks and is tasteless.

Lecithin

Lecithin is a supplement that has soap-like qualities that act as an emulsifying agent. Its presence in the blood may tend to dissolve cholesterol deposits. These deposits can inhibit or totally block the flow of blood to the cells of the brain and cause them to die. Therefore, it is essential that the small blood vessels be kept open and clear. Lecithin can help greatly in this respect. Lecithin is available in liquid, capsule, and granules—the latter being the most potent and economical form.

Breakfast—A Brain Bonanza

We must remember that good nutrition begins with good food, and the best place to begin any nutrition regime is at breakfast. The human machine needs fuel to run on and breakfast is the first chance we have to "fuel up." We should never begin the day without a good, highly-nutritious breakfast. We should have at least one top-grade protein and a constructive carbohydrate. If we are not comfortable with a large breakfast, let's begin with a very small one. Once we see the benefits that good food in the morning brings us throughout the day, it will soon become a habit.

Are You Ready to Begin?

Let's get started on the road back to solid health. We will begin as all journeys must begin—by seeking first the kingdom of God. We put God first in all we do. As long as we keep God first, we know we cannot fail.

Next we deny the inevitability of senility. Senility is not "natural." Nobody has to become senile just because he has lived a certain number of years. Age is chronological not pathological. Age itself can cause nothing. Our years are a man-made measurement indicating the number of times we have circled the sun. We must *never* be limited by that.

And let's not forget that the brain is part of the body and we must choose only the finest foods to rebuild that body. When we realize that we are temples of God, we will desire only the finest foods to renovate and restore our temples.

The answer to senility lies in our nourishing the life force with thoughts of God and in our obedience to the laws of God. When we really begin to do the former, we will automatically be led to do the latter. And when we do it all, how can we fail?

Happy, Healthy Hearts

On all the Earth there is no motor—no pump—as wonderfully constructed as the human heart. It is the strongest of all body structures and endowed with incredible endurance to keep it operating continuously. Night and day, year after year, this mighty motor pumps the red life-stream through our blood vessels. It is dauntless, full of valor, fronting terrible adversities to keep us alive. We do not yet know the true physiological potential of the human heart, but we do know that as the center of love in the body it has no limits.

The heart has traditionally been the symbol of the love nature—the feeling nature. From the Bible to modern day love songs, from ". . . *you shall love the Lord your God with all your heart, and with all your soul, and with all your might*" (Deut. 6:5) to "I Left My Heart in San Francisco"— the heart has always been identified with our emotions, particularly love.

Because this phenomenal organ is so crucial to life itself, it must be given optimum care, respect, and praise. It goes about its job of supplying us with life without our being consciously aware of it. It knows exactly what to do and how to do it. Perhaps nowhere else in the body temple does the Creator manifest Himself in such an obvious manner as He does in the heart. With each mighty beat He sends forth love and life to our tissues in an almost compulsive rhythm. The creative life force cannot help itself from surging forward toward more and better life. It knows no other plan.

But we must do *our* share. We were given the highest

of all gifts in creation—the gift of life. It is up to us to receive that gift, work with it, and obey the laws which govern it. There is no other way. When we do our share, God can always be counted on to do His. *And by this we know that he abides in us, by the Spirit which he has given us.* (I John 3:24)

Much has been written about the metaphysical meanings of the heart. The cardiac plexus is generally regarded as the love center of the body. Charles Fillmore makes many references to the heart as being the great equalizer of the flow of life in the body just as love is the great harmonizer of the thoughts of the mind.

If our hearts are filled with bitterness, hate, and other negative emotions, our bodies often manifest heart disease and other circulatory problems. That is why Mr. Fillmore wrote: *Our dominant thoughts about love will show forth in the heart center and establish there a general character. The loves and hates of the mind are precipitated to this ganglionic receptacle of thought and crystallized there. Its substance is sensitive, tremulous, and volatile. What we love or what we hate builds cells of joy or pain in the cardiac plexus.*

The nerves around the heart are very sensitive to thoughts of fear, anxiety, and hatred. Nothing stresses the heart as much as these incapacitating emotions, with the result that the heart is held in a vise-like grip of negativism that often produces a physical heart symptom of some type.

We must look first to our love nature whenever we seek to help the heart. We must be kind, loving, and forgiving in order to let the life force flow unobstructedly throughout our bodies. . . . *be kind to one another, tenderhearted, forgiving one another, as God in Christ forgave you.* (Eph. 4:32)

We should meditate each day on the idea of divine love, concentrating on our love center in the heart. This opens the channel for the love current and allows the old crystallized hatreds to be broken up and swept away. This is a most important consideration for anyone who would have a healthy heart, for a troubled heart cannot be a sound one. *"Let not your hearts be troubled, neither let them be afraid."* (John 14:27)

The first rule then in preventing or overcoming heart trouble is that of making love and peace a habit in our lives. *. . . let the peace of Christ rule in your hearts . . . .* (Col. 3:15) This is the basis of all heart health and must be practiced faithfully in order that we might let this mighty motor express itself perfectly, continuing its matchless performance of bringing us life.

Enemies of the Heart

The inscrutable heart, miraculous and splendid as it is, is not without its enemies. There are those factors that work against the heart, seeking to tear it down and destroy it. We should all be aware of these malefactors and do our best to avoid them.

The major foes of the heart are these: stress, tobacco, alcohol, narcotics, sugar, white flour, all junk foods, vitamin and mineral deficiencies, and lack of exercise. There are many forms of stress, including all eight of the other heart enemies. In addition, tension arising from human relationship situations, employment circumstances, and all sorts of other pressures we encounter in our world can lead to stress on the body and the soul. We have to learn to handle these from our Christ nature, always turning within to find poise and peacefulness. In this way we do not allow these would-be stresses to become part of our lives and thus we deprive them of their potential danger.

Life Is Motion

Oh, how the heart loves exercise. It is a muscle, after all, and muscles must be used or they atrophy and degenerate. Regular exercise to increase the pulse rate is excellent for toning up the heart. If you are under the care of a physician, he can guide you in this important activity. There are countless records of cardiac patients who have restored normal function to their hearts through proper exercise.

Brisk walking is an excellent exercise for the heart and circulatory system. Begin with a short distance and gradually increase it. You will soon amaze yourself at the increase in your stamina and sense of well-being. Before long you will be briskly walking several miles daily and feeling great doing it.

Bicycle riding also is good exercise. So is swimming. Exercise must be done regularly if it is to be beneficial to the heart. The "weekend athlete" who pushes his body to the limit after a sedentary week in the office is doing himself much more harm than good. The benefits lie in the regularity.

It is important to give consideration to a regular exercise plan. Don't overdo—don't force and exhaust the body. Use good judgment always. But keep in mind that the body *must* move if the heart is to survive. Good exercise can strengthen the heart tissues, making them more durable and efficient. Motion is basic to life. Incorporate some form of exercise into your healthy heart program. The strong, steady beat of your heart will be saying, "Thank you, thank you, thank you!"

Dr. Irving Oyle noted in his book "The Healing Mind" that at a recent cardiology conference it was revealed that too many patients were choosing to undergo coronary bypass operations rather than change their life-styles, which were leading to the coronary disease. *Most people,* states Dr. Oyle, *would rather submit to an operation that promises to cure them quickly, even at the risk of death, than lose weight, give up smoking, and slow down.* These people are trying to take shortcuts to health, ignoring the old heart foes that threaten to weaken and destroy them, and they are not facing the truth that the law of cause and effect is immutable. They think an operation will somehow suspend the law, but it just does not work that way.

We must be true to our body temples and the life force within them. This means avoiding the heart enemies and doing our best for our temples. We have already discussed the roles of love, peace, and exercise. It is time to study the nutritional requirements of a healthy heart.

Good Food for Good Hearts

Strong hearts cannot be built without good amounts of top-grade protein. Each meal should contain at least one protein food. Proteins are the best building materials for the body temple.

The foods we eat literally become heart tissue. They are incorporated into the body. Therefore, our health is directly related to the quality of the food we ingest. The great biochemist Dr. Roger J. Williams in his highly recommended book "Nutrition Against Disease" has this to say: *People may think that when they eat candy or drink an alcoholic beverage they will make up for it later by eating good wholesome food. It doesn't work that way.* A foe is a foe and the damage is always done.

Dr. Williams relates his own dramatic recovery from heart disease through good nutrition and exercise. He goes on to say: *All hearts require vastly better protection and maintenance than they are getting. . . . Nothing is so im-*

117

*portant in the micro-environment of the living cells in heart
and blood vessels and elsewhere as the assortment of nutrient substances in which these cells are continually
bathed. . . . Nutrition has come to be of medical concern
with heart disease. . . . It is cellular nutrition that needs
attention.*

Cellular nutrition is what we must devote ourselves to if
we want good hearts. In addition to the top-grade protein,
we need the constructive (not destructive) carbohydrates:
fresh fruits, fresh vegetables, and whole grains (including
sugarless whole grain breads). If we need to sweeten something, we should use small amounts of honey, blackstrap
molasses, or pure maple syrup. (Artificial sweeteners are
not foods and do not belong in the body temple.)

The heart is not helped by junk foods and begs us not
to introduce them into our divine tissues. Our first concern
in selecting a food should always be whether it will help
build health, not whether it will please a few taste buds that
have been perverted by a history of bad nutrition. Sugar,
white flour—and all the products made from them—are
definitely out if health is to be in.

We need some good oil each day. The choice of good
cold-pressed (actually mechanically pressed) oil will be very
beneficial. Safflower, corn, sunflower, and sesame are all
good oils. Refrigerate them after opening. Wheat germ oil is
excellent for the heart and can be taken in capsule form if
preferred. Note that it takes four capsules of the twenty
minim size to equal about one teaspoonful of the oil.

What About Cholesterol?

For those who are wondering about cholesterol, let's
take time right now to examine the facts. Many studies have
been done which prove that the much-maligned egg is

seldom the culprit in elevated cholesterol levels. This from Roger Williams, who reminds us that cholesterol is necessary for our bodies and is good, not bad, in its proper place: *How can this depositing of cholesterol be prevented? The most obvious answer is "consume less cholesterol." Superficially, this sounds like a good suggestion; actually it is a poor one. Most of our good foods contain substantial amounts of cholesterol, and if we try to eliminate cholesterol consumption we sacrifice good nutrition . . . . Anyone who deliberately avoids cholesterol in his diet may be inadvertently courting heart disease . . . . The evidence points to the conclusion that good nutrition, if it is really good, prevents cholesterol deposits from forming, even when our cholesterol consumption is moderately high. We must remember that cholesterol is made with our bodies, and that this "homemade" cholesterol can be deposited in the arteries of a person who consumes no cholesterol at all.* He further states that eating no cholesterol foods can possibly create a build-up in the body. *A better answer to the problem of cholesterol deposits may be this: consume more lecithin. It is known that lecithin . . . is a powerful emulsifying agent, and its presence in the blood tends to dissolve cholesterol deposits.*

This excerpt from "A Physician's Handbook on Orthomolecular Medicine" is worth noting: *It has been found that adding sugar to the diet of both men and animals will raise the blood cholesterol, and adding fiber will lower it.* (Fruits, vegetables, and especially whole grains contain good amounts of fiber. Bran is almost pure fiber and the addition to the diet of one or two teaspoonful of this harmless bulk two or three times a day may be a good idea. (If the bran presents a gas problem, cut down on the amount you use until your body gets accustomed to it.)

Writing in "Executive Health," Dr. Mark D. Altschule

tells us: . . . *if all you want to know is whether so many of your favorite foods, such as eggs, that contain cholesterol increase your risk of heart disease, they do not!*

The textbook "Nutrition in Health and Disease" discusses the role of ascorbic acid (vitamin C) in the elimination of cholesterol. The liver converts the cholesterol to bile acids which are excreted. Adequate amounts of vitamin C are required for this process.

What is all this saying? What does it mean to us? In essence it means to eat properly. It means consume more lecithin (about one to three tablespoonsful of the granules each day. It takes about fourteen or fifteen of the nineteen-grain capsules to equal the potency of a tablespoonful, so the granules are more practical!). It means avoid sugar. It means get plenty of fiber (bulk) in the form of fresh vegetables and fruits and grains or unprocessed bran, if necessary. And it means taking an adequate amount of vitamin C. Many scientists estimate that between 1,000 and 5,000 milligrams are adequate, others estimate up to 10,000 milligrams. We each must find out how much is best for us.

We cannot determine our individual needs by basing them on the needs of a statistical "average." We must always work gently with the life force within us to get the "feel" about a nutrient. We can develop body wisdom only when we tune ourselves in to this life force and its needs.

Vitamin and Mineral Friends

One of the enemies of the heart that was mentioned earlier was vitamin and mineral deficiencies. Good supplementation should be included in our plan for a healthy heart.

Plenty of complete B complex (eleven B vitamins) is essential to the heart. Vitamin C has already been mentioned in its role with cholesterol. Biochemist Irwin Stone, after more than forty years of research on vitamin C, reached this conclusion: *All of this provocative and sugges-tive research . . . indicates that the simple ingestion of three to five grams [3,000 to 5,000 milligrams] of ascorbic acid a day in several spaced doses may be sufficient . . . to prevent the high incidence of heart disease and strokes.* He added that those who are treated with vitamin C after suffering heart attacks and strokes stand a much better chance of survival and recovery.

Vitamin E is another key vitamin. It can be an impor-tant factor in the prevention of heart disease and in the re-habilitation of the heart. If you are interested in the various roles vitamin E plays in the cardiovascular system, you would benefit by reading "Vitamin E for Ailing and Healthy Hearts," by Wilfrid E. Shute, MD, of the Shute Foundation for Medical Research in Canada. Dr. Shute and his brother Evan, also a physician, have done much of the pioneering work with this versatile vitamin. They report that vitamin E will . . . *not only dissolve clots, but circulating in the blood of a healthy individual will prevent thrombi from forming.* The book, a result of the extensive clinical research done by the Shute brothers, makes this statement: *By now it is possi-ble to say with complete assurance that alpha tocopherol [vitamin E] is a thoroughly tried and tested therapeutic agent, unusually successful in its results and with its effect so well defined that it can be used with precision by any com-petent physician.*

When using vitamin E, we always begin with small amounts: 50 or 100 International Units (I.U.) per day for a month or so. Then we double the dose for another month, and then do the same every month. In this way we build up our dosage gradually, observing the results as we go. While most people end up taking between 400 to 800 I.U.'s of vitamin E daily, it would be advisable to read Dr. Shute's book to be able to more effectively tailor your dosage to your own needs. (Those with serious heart problems should *first* consult with their physicians.)

Minerals have an important role to play in the health of the heart. Calcium, magnesium, and potassium are the major minerals we should present to our bodies if we want our hearts to keep beating properly. These are electrolytes, and their presence in the heart is critical to its health.

Minerals are found in good foods, so we begin with a diet rich in these elements. Potassium, for instance, is found in good amounts in many fresh fruits and vegetables. Green leafy vegetables usually contain magnesium in good amounts. Milk and cheeses are among the best sources of calcium. But we may not be able to obtain the required amounts of these vital minerals—especially calcium—from our foods.

Calcium is difficult for the body to absorb. We seem to have trouble obtaining sufficient amounts of this major mineral from our foods and may have to look to calcium supplements if we are seeking optimum health. Many types of calcium are available. Liquid calcium tablets or bone meal or calcium lactate are good, as are many others.

Small amounts of magnesium and potassium supplements might prove valuable also. Perhaps a mineral complex tablet containing magnesium, potassium, calcium, and all the other important minerals would be helpful.

The heart also has need of certain trace minerals, such as chromium and selenium. These important minerals are in good supply in the fine foods that God has given us, especially whole grains, organ meats, nuts, and seeds.

Through following a good nutritional regime, one that supplies all the elements necessary for happy, healthy hearts, you can find yourself . . . *singing and making melody to the Lord with all your heart. . . .* (Eph. 5:19) It will be natural for you to joyously praise God for the health you now experience.

To summarize, let us take a quick look at what the *ideal* program for happy, healthy hearts would be.

1. We first seek God—the Christ within—and make contact with our love centers, letting them flood our hearts and minds with healing, forgiving power. *. . . let the hearts of those who seek the Lord rejoice!* (Psalms 105:3)

2. Embark on a good, regular program of physical exercise.

3. Eliminate as much stress as possible from your life. (When you succeed in attaining the first part of the program, this will happen automatically.)

4. Avoid tobacco, alcohol, white flour, sugar, and all junk foods.

5. Obtain top-grade protein, constructive carbohydrates, and a good oil at each meal, making sure of sufficient fiber in the diet.

6. Supplement the diet with complete B complex, vitamin C, vitamin E, calcium, magnesium, and potassium.

This six-point program is not a temporary plan. It is a way of life that will result after we change our consciousness—the place where it *all* starts! Our hearts are symbols of the love of God, working within our body temples to bring us life. Let us cherish our precious hearts, observing all the God-given laws by which they function.

If your heart is strong and healthy, give thanks and do everything in your power to keep it that way. If your heart needs regenerating, bless it and do everything in your power to restore it to its rightful perfection. Work with the laws of Spirit, soul, and body; remain faithful to the loving life force pulsing within you . . . *until the day dawns and the morning star rises in your hearts.* (II Peter 1:19) On that day will your soul sing with God's melody of life as you joyfully step to the rhythm of your own happy, healthy heart.

Life for the Lungs

Air—the breath of life! We cannot exist without it. We can go for a short time without water and a much longer time without food. But in order to remain alive, we need air continuously.

Our wonderful lungs operate on a system of denials and affirmations. They breathe in life-giving oxygen, which is then picked up by the blood and circulated throughout the body in a grand affirmation of our being. They then remove the waste product carbon dioxide from the blood and breathe it out in a great denial of the negative and useless. And this marvel of breathing is done not only in the lungs but within each cell of the body as it breathes in new life and releases the old. Truly nothing could be more symbolic of life itself than breathing. *Thus says the Lord God to these bones: Behold, I will cause breath to enter you, and you shall live.* (Ezek. 37:5)

Breathing is even more than a physiological activity, however. It is the symbol of spiritual inspiration. Jesus breathed upon His disciples and said to them, *"Receive the Holy Spirit."* (John 20:22) Charles Fillmore refers to this in *Mysteries of Genesis: God is breathing His breath through man's being, cleansing the blood stream, and filling his whole being with spiritual understanding.*

As we breathe in life, we are made aware of our oneness with God. And breathing makes us equally aware of our oneness with the entire universe as we breathe out life, sending it forth to become part of the ethers. In his book "Your Power To Be," J. Sig Paulson uses these words:

Breathing reveals our unity with all other creatures (atoms, plants, animals)—when we breathe in, we are drawing on an element to which all have contributed and when we breathe out we are ourselves making a contribution to the universal atmosphere. This reveals the law of "giving and receiving" or the principle of circulation on which all life form is dependent.

If our lungs are not sound and functioning according to the grand design of the perfect body temple, we should examine our lives from the spiritual aspect and see what we can come up with metaphysically. Catherine Ponder, in "The Healing Secret of the Ages," suggests that diseases of the lungs and chest area are often a result of one's disturbances in his affections and love nature. The only way to ascertain the real cause metaphysically is to meditate—go within for the answer.

All the work must be done within, of course. We know that each cell is an intelligent being that responds to our thoughts, words, and emotions. That is why Myrtle Fillmore went to all the areas of her body and spoke words of Truth, strength, and life to them. She asked their forgiveness for the foolishness and ignorance with which she had treated them in the past. And it worked!

In *Mysteries of John* Charles Fillmore discussed the marvelous workings of the lungs: *If your lung capacity is not equal to the purification of your blood, increase it by declaring the law of active life. Anemic blood may be made vigorous and virile by daily centering the attention in the lungs and affirming them to be spiritual; and under the perpetual inflow of new life and the outflow of old life the lungs will do your will.*

All disease and negative conditions begin in the mind. There is something in the consciousness that is causing these troublesome manifestations in the body. It is to the mind that we must look for the causes, correcting them by aligning ourselves with our spiritual perfection.

The Smoking Syndrome

Many people attribute lung problems, especially the condition labeled as emphysema, to the habit of smoking. And this is frequently the case. But while we certainly need to give up the use of tobacco if we are seeking perfection, we must learn to look beyond the physical practice to the state of consciousness that is responsible for the desire to smoke in the first place.

We always must turn our attention back within ourselves to get at the real cause of things and to resolve them. So, if you have any lung problem, there would seem to be work waiting to be done in the consciousness.

Let's spend a few moments on the very obvious villain—smoking. It has been said that all of our illnesses are self-inflicted. If we believe in the law of mind action, we can accept this as true. However, it is not only in the mental realm that God's laws can be violated. If we disregard the laws of creation—those physical laws that govern our body temples—we will find that our health will weaken.

It is our responsibility to know these physical (yet divine) laws and practice obeying them. *Teach me, O Lord, the way of thy statutes; and I will keep it to the end. Give me understanding, that I may keep thy law and observe it with my whole heart.* (Psalms 119:33, 34) Putting poisonous smoke in contact with the beautiful pink tissues of the lungs is not one of God's laws! And no amount of affirmations or prayers to the contrary will ameliorate the terrible effects of such a practice. If every action is actually a prayer, indicating our true belief about ourselves and our Creator, then every time we smoke we are offering up a colossal denial of life and the divinity within us.

In *Atom-Smashing Power of Mind,* Charles Fillmore admonishes us that we must begin to obey the laws of the body temple: *The fact is that we have reached a point in race evolution where we are forced to give attention to the refinement of our body. Our religion has too long taught that the body is dust and ashes and that it is its destiny to die and be left to the worms. The deterioration of our body cells must be arrested and a new and more powerful life force injected into the physical organism.*

And how can we inject this *new and powerful life force* into our organisms if we are injecting black, noxious tobacco fumes into them? It doesn't make sense, does it? The body wants more than anything else to be whole and sound, and it struggles against all kinds of odds to supply us with life. It is amazing, actually, what the body will put up with in its determination to survive.

Medical science attests to this phenomenon of the incredible determination of the life force. In his book "The Body Is the Hero," Ronald J. Glasser, MD describes this drive: *Our body will take care of itself if given the slightest chance. It already has the best of nature within it and will survive if we will only let it, if we give it just half the chance it has given and continues to give each of us.*

Yet we refuse so often to give our bodies this chance. We continue to smoke, eat abominably, and over-stress ourselves, obtaining little or no exercise. Even when our bodies are rebelling with disease and discomfort, we insist upon pursuing the same old suicidal ways. Dr. Irving Oyle, in "The Healing Mind," remarks about this stubborn foolishness: *People tend to cling tenaciously to their habit pattern, even in the face of violent somatic (body) opposition.*

If you are facing emphysema or other lung or bronchial ailments and are still smoking, you are undoubtedly aware of the collision course on which you travel. But it is a fact that no one will relinquish the habit of smoking until he is really "ready" to do it—until he has relinquished it from his consciousness and the full awareness of what he has been doing finally dawns on him. At this point he will no longer regard himself, no longer think of himself, as "a smoker." It will be gone from his consciousness and, therefore, soon gone from his outer physical expression. But until that time arrives, the habit will always be there to contend with and fight.

Myrtle Said It Best!

If you are trying to give up smoking, here is a most powerful and graphic quote from Myrtle Fillmore that might just have an impact on you. Read it slowly, thoughtfully, and allow your imagination to visualize these highly descriptive words: *I can't quite see the picture of [Jesus] with a cigarette or cigar hanging from His mouth, or even between His fingers. I can't see a cloud of smoke enveloping His head, or pouring from His lips. And I can't quite imagine His laying a cigarette on the table or tossing it to the ground, before stretching forth His hand to bless and to heal one who comes to Him in faith.*

"Yes, but that was Jesus," you say. "I am not He." Oh, but you contain the Christ just as surely as did Jesus. And are we not told that Jesus is our Way-Shower, giving us the pattern by which we are to become perfect, even as our Father in heaven is perfect? Next time you reach for a cigarette (or whatever vehicle of smoke you employ), try rereading those vivid words of Myrtle and perhaps something will begin to change. And what a great day of victory that day will be!

Methods of Improvement

Of course, the change must be initiated in our consciousness. We must first of all *want* to be well. We must *desire* the perfection that we were meant to be. After this desire is firmly established as part of our thought pattern, there is much that can be done to help lung problems—including emphysema. Through correction of diet, the use of certain vitamin and mineral supplements, and a program of fresh air, sunshine, and regular exercise, these weakened, flaccid tissues can be regenerated into the strong, resilient ones they were designed to be.

First, since the lungs, like the rest of the body, are largely protein in substance, we must be certain of a good intake of protein foods if we want to rebuild this tissue. Eggs, milk, cheese, fish, fowl, and lean meat are the sources of complete protein.

Next, we need only the best carbohydrates. Eliminate *completely* the sugars, junk foods, and refined carbohydrates from your diet. Instead, use only fresh fruits, vegetables, whole grains (including whole-grain breads, if you desire) and small amounts of honey, blackstrap molasses, and pure maple syrup if you must sweeten something. The destructive carbohydrates—and the list is endless—litter the body with toxins and alter chemistry, blocking chances of regeneration. The more pure and natural the food, the easier it is for the body temple to utilize it effectively.

We also need some good cold-pressed oil each day. For use on salads and in cooking, a good-tasting oil like safflower or corn oil is a fine choice. Buy the finest available—one without perservatives would be best.

Minerals and Vitamins

Calcium is a mineral required by the lungs to build integrity and strength into their tissues. Therefore, a good calcium supplement is in order. Perhaps the liquid calcium in capsule form would work best for you, since the body seems to absorb it fairly easily. Take several capsules at each meal and even before bed.

When it comes to vitamins, let us assume that you are taking a good multiple formula containing ample amounts of all of the vitamins, especially the B complex. Remember, the body is manifesting a physical problem, so don't be afraid to give it all the help it needs.

Our next consideration would be some extra vitamin A to strengthen the integrity of the special cells of the lungs. These cells are highly specialized epithelial cells which God has designed to allow life-giving oxygen to enter our bloodstreams and suffocating carbon dioxide to leave. Any impairment in the structure of these cells interferes with our oxygen supply and interferes with our perfect expression of the indwelling life force.

In order to prevent the oxidation of Vitamin A (and also of the polyunsaturated fat in cod liver oil) a supplemental amount of vitamin E is important. This wonderful vitamin performs a plethora of important biochemical actions in our bodies; but in a program of lung health, its most important function is its interaction with vitamin A.

No program of bodily renewal would be complete without the assurance of enough vitamin C in the diet. This is truly one of the "superstars" of nutrition. Among the numerous tasks that vitamin C performs, none is more important than its use in the manufacture of collagen—the "cement" that holds cells together. Add to this its role in cellular respiration, its use in proper absorption of iron, its anti-atherogenic effects, and the many, many more jobs it performs, and you can see the need for optimum amounts of this special vitamin.

And what is an optimum amount? Many authorities recommend between 1,000 and 5,000 milligrams daily of vitamin C. Some say at least 10,000 milligrams should be taken daily. We will need, of course, to decide for ourselves just what is optimum.

Work your way up in the amounts you take and see how much your body requires for its best functioning. Along with the vitamin C (ascorbic acid) it is beneficial to take bio-flavonoids, which are part of the vitamin C family. Vitamin C and bioflavonoids can be purchased in one tablet or separately.

Another product that is very beneficial to weakened tissues is lecithin. This is a food substance, available in granules (the most potent form), and it can be added to salads, soups, vegetables, juices, protein drinks, or taken from a spoon. One or more tablespoonsful a day could prove to be helpful. It can be purchased in a health food store.

Exercise is a vital part of any health program—and health is what we are after, isn't it? It is important that we exercise our lungs because they were designed to move effortlessly. The human body, unlike a machine, wears out from *non*-use.

We can exercise our lungs with breathing exercises. Deep breathing helps us to utilize our entire lung capacity. (Most of the time we are using only a small portion of our capacity.) There are yoga exercises that help the breathing, and there are other types of breathing exercises as well. Don't overdo. Gently coax the body, never force. But do practice these breathing exercises if you want to improve.

Walking, swimming, and cycling are good for the lungs

as are many other mild exercises. You can find an activity that suits you and make it a habit—a habit for health.

We Have a Choice

The day is not far distant when humanity will realize that biologically it is faced with a choice between suicide and adoration. These are the words of Pierre Teilhard de Chardin in his book "The Divine Milieu." Let us stop plundering our body temples by smoking, eating harmful foods, and not exercising. Let us turn away from the suicidal bent of these practices and become aware of the miracle of life we truly are.

With this awareness will come the adoration of which Teilhard speaks. Our hearts will be filled with praise and joy and our lungs will once again be able to fill easily and effortlessly with the breath of life.

Abolishing Alcoholism

There is perhaps no malady that touches the lives of the entire family of the one afflicted as does alcoholism. And there is no malady so consistently referred by physicians to lay people for treatment! It is surely a unique affliction. For those manifesting alcoholism, and for their loved ones suffering along with them, it may seem preposterous to suggest that alcoholism can be overcome. And yet it can be, for in God's realm there are no alcoholics!

It is easy for those suffering through this malady to forget this Truth, because alcoholics are not made in a few weeks. It usually takes many years of drinking and nutritional abuse before alcoholism emerges. Although such people may not admit it, they know they have a drinking problem. During this time, they feel guilt, self-condemnation, self-pity, anger—the gamut of human emotions. They feel "in bondage to the bottle." They feel that it is their lot to be weak and unable to refrain from drinking. Alcoholics are not sure they are loved by their families or friends. But worse than that, they feel separated from God. They are not sure that God loves them. It is this feeling of separation from God—from good—that leads to the ills in any of our lives.

First Phase of Renewal

In order to overcome alcoholism, there must be renewed attention directed to the three phases of our being: Spirit, soul, and body. As always, we will want to begin with the Spirit phase.

The Spirit aspect of our being is our eternal, unchanging, divine pattern. It is our indestructible design for perfection. Any manifestation we are now showing that is not in concert with this perfection is false and must be purged from our lives. Perfection is part of our grand design. Jesus referred to this when He said: . . . *"Is it not written in your law, 'I said, Ye are gods'?"* (John 10:34)

It is essential, therefore, that you think of yourself as manifesting the design that is your potential. You must never believe you are anything but *perfect* in potential. Release forever from your mind that you are an alcoholic. You may be manifesting a very serioius drinking problem to be sure, and know that it is temporary and that it is *not* the true you—it is not your nature to be an alcoholic. *It is your nature to be a perfect creation of God, and that only!*

We seek our perfection by first seeking God. We can overcome nothing without first directing our lives to Him. If we feel we have been proceeding in the wrong direction, let us turn our lives around. It is *never* too late, for God is quintessential forgiveness.

Role of the Soul

The soul is our consciousness. It is what we have apprehended out of Spirit. It is our individual awareness of our existence. It encompasses the entire mind. The soul is pivotal—it can turn its thinking inward where it will receive impressions from Spirit or outward where impressions will be gleaned through the five senses. Obviously the more we turn our minds inward the closer we will mirror our perfect design. To base our thoughts and feelings on such imperfect sentinels as the five senses is folly. In the case of alcoholism, it is to believe that a certain chemical substance has dominion over our lives! It is to believe that when two atoms of carbon, six atoms of hydrogen, and one atom of oxygen arrange themselves in a certain structure, which chemists have named ethyl alcohol, we must then be in bondage to these atoms. Imagine giving a chemical dominion over our lives! Let us get our thoughts turned inward and take our direction from our Christ center, which is the real link we have with God.

And, if we are to help someone who seems to be in bondage to alcohol, it is our duty to see him as a perfect creation of God and not as an alcoholic. We can do nothing better for that person than to see him as perfect and know that he has within him the seed of his own salvation from alcoholism. What *we* cannot do for him the Spirit of God in him can do and will do when we don't inhibit its expression with fear, worry, anxiety, and condemnation.

Physical Realm

This brings us to the third phase of being: body. This is the vehicle through which Spirit and soul express. When the soul is using all the divine ideas in the right way, the body sings a song of love to the universe. However, unhappy, anxious, fearful, and chaotic states of mind will make the body turn from its divine design and will cause suffering.

The body is a chemical compound. The thoughts we think and the food we eat affect that chemistry. Discordant thoughts will yield discordant body chemistry. Discordant food will yield discordant body chemistry, and discordant body chemistry will yield "sickness," including alcoholism. It is elementary. We are dealing with the law of cause and effect. We must obey *all* God's laws.

There is no hierarchy of laws in the universe. The laws

of nutrition are just as much a part of God's laws of healing and wholeness as are any others. However, it is essential to note that there can never be a *permanent* healing without a corresponding permanent change in consciousness. With this in mind, let us investigate the nutritional aspects of alcoholism.

Nutrition is a crucial factor—for or against alcoholism. In an experiment done with laboratory rats, the animals were fed a nutritious ration and, for a beverage, had a choice of water or alcohol mixed with water. Most chose only water, but a few would occasionally sip from the mixture of alcohol and water. The experimenters then changed the ration so that it had less nutrients. When this happened, more of the rats chose the alcohol mixture. As the diets were made to become more and more deficient, more and more rats chose the alcoholic mixture. Finally, when the diet was extremely deficient, all the animals lost their body wisdom and consumed the alcohol mixture at a very high level.

When the diet was changed to a complete, well-fortified one, supplemented with vitamins and minerals, the rats all regained their body wisdom and turned away from alcohol consumption.

In a similar experiment, all the laboratory rats became alcoholic when their good diet was changed to that of the typical American teenage diet! When coffee was added to this already poor nutrition, the rats became even worse drinkers!

These and many other experiments have led one of America's greatest scientists, biochemist Roger J. Williams, to state: *I will . . . herewith positively assert that no one who follows good nutritional patterns will ever become an alcoholic.* Many researchers of alcoholism agree with Dr. Williams. They note that compulsive alcohol consumption is often accompanied by aversion or indifference to food. This indicates that the part of the brain that controls the appetite is out of order. Dr. Williams notes: *Whatever else may happen to consumers of alcohol only those whose appetite mechanisms are deranged become alcoholics.* He notes that the drinking of alcohol tends to make mediocre or poor nutrition even poorer. It does this in two ways: First, alcohol crowds out of the diet many important nutrients which the body must have to function properly. And secondly, alcohol itself is poisonous to human cells. It pollutes our inner environment.

In fact, one of the cofounders of Alcoholics Anonymous extolled the virtues of good nutrition, supplemental vitamins, and high-protein diets in the control of alcoholism.

With these facts in mind, let us now see how we can utilize the wonderful foods God has given us to build bodies that will more fully express our divine blueprint, bodies that will have only *one* craving—that of abundant life.

Laws of Nutrition

Any nutritional regime designed to build or rebuild the body temple must have protein as its primary consideration. The life force within us uses protein as the building blocks with which it fashions human tissues. There can be no building without protein. (See chapter two, page 17, for a listing of top-grade proteins and carbohydrates.)

Many investigators regard a high-protein diet as the nutritional key to rehabilitation for the alcoholic. When one considers that hypoglycemia (low blood sugar) is almost always involved in alcoholism and that high-protein diets are essential to the hypoglycemic, one can begin to see why protein is so important. A generous serving of one or more of the top-grade proteins at each meal is a must.

Regular ingestion of the constructive carbohydrates is essential. The life-giving carbohydrates are fresh fruits (apples, bananas, peaches, melons, pears, and others), fresh vegetables (squashes, green beans, potatoes, carrots, salad greens, tomatoes, and much more), and whole grains (brown rice, whole-grain buckwheat, wheat, rye, barley, millet, oats, and others, including breads made from these whole grains). These carbohydrates abound with the life force.

If a sweetener must be used, try very small amounts of honey (tupelo honey is best), blackstrap molasses, or pure maple syrup. Don't overdo these sweeteners; they can present problems if taken in large amounts.

No nutritional regime is complete without oils. Everybody has a need for essential fatty acids, especially one called linoleic acid, and most good vegetable oils present the body with these essentials. In the case of alcoholics this need is particularly acute. There is much evidence that those suffering from alcoholism have special need of linoleic acid because of its role in the body's manufacturing of something called gamma-linoleic acid (GLA). This GLA in turn is crucial to the manufacturing of a certain family of prostaglandins—those powerful chemicals found in every cell, which regulate the way in which every organ works. It has been shown that people with low levels of certain prostaglandins are likely to become alcoholics.

Oils high in linoleic acid are safflower, sunflower, corn, sesame, and soy. Purchase them raw and untreated containing no preservatives. Use them on salads, baked potatoes, vegetables, and in Better Butter (see chapter two, page 24, for recipe). After opening, be sure to refrigerate the oils.

Nuts and seeds, in addition to being wonderful snacks,

are also sources of good oils. They should become a part of our daily nutrition. Always eat them raw and unsalted.

But for people who drink alcohol, these oils may not be enough because the more alcohol consumed the less able the body is to convert linoleic acid to GLA. Chronic alcohol consumption completely blocks the ability of the body to do this! Because of their inability to make this conversion and thus the crucial prostaglandins, those who drink alcohol—and especially chronic drinkers—would be very wise to seek a direct source of GLA. Such a source (and one of the only food sources) is the oil extracted from the seeds of the evening primrose. Dr. David F. Horrobin is one of the world's leading authorities on essential fatty acids and prostaglandins and an expert on their effects in alcoholism. He states that essential fatty acids (found most abundantly in vegetable oils) and, in the case of chronic drinkers, primrose seed oil, can . . . *relieve hangovers and post drinking depressions.* . . . He goes on to say that he believes that these . . . *will prove a major advance in helping alcoholics to withdraw from alcohol.*

He suggests taking from four to eight 0.5 gram capsules daily of the evening primrose oil. (If you do drink, he suggests an additional four capsules with a glass of water before retiring and four upon arising.)

That covers the nutritionally essential foods. Good nutrition begins with good foods, not with vitamins and minerals. For an alcoholic, a bad diet with plenty of vitamins and minerals is still a bad diet. A good diet without extra vitamins and minerals is still a good diet. But a good diet *with* supplemental vitamins and minerals may be a better diet!

In studying the literature dealing with alcoholism, one is struck with the plethora of nutritional deficiencies that alcoholics can manifest. Of course, in light of their long

history of atrocious eating habits, this should not be sur-
prising. Implicated among the deficiencies are most of the B
complex vitamins and vitamin C, along with such minerals
as magnesium, zinc, and many more (and, in fact, all of
these specific vitamins and minerals are needed by the body
to make prostaglandins!).

With this in mind, much care should be given to selecting a potent, complete multiple vitamin-mineral supplement
containing high amounts of all eleven of the B complex vitamins, good amounts of vitamin C, plus vitamins A, D, and
E, and all the essential minerals. This will assure at least a
minimum intake if used daily. However, we should not
assume that this minimum supplementation will be enough.
Until we have rebuilt our bodies and healed all our nutritional injuries, we may need many times the normal
amounts of certain nutrients! If we present the body with an
abundance of nutrients, it will choose what it needs and reject what it does not. If we present the body with insufficient
amounts, it obviously does not have this option. A good
multiple vitamin-mineral supplement is an excellent place to
start.

In addition to being a drug, ethanol (alcohol) is also—
strictly speaking—a high calorie food. In any dose, of
course, it is a toxic poison: inTOXICation! Nevertheless, in
no matter what quantities it is consumed it still must be
metabolized. Since alcohol contains only "naked" calories,
just food energy and no vitamins or minerals, the body must
use its own nutrients to metabolize it. The vitamins most
essential for this type of metabolism are the vitamins of the
B complex family. Those B complex vitamins found to be
especially important in the case of alcoholics are thiamine
(B1), riboflavin (B2), pyridoxine (B6), niacin (sometimes
called B3), and folic acid. Since the B complex vitamins
(and vitamin C) cannot be stored in the body, it is impera-

tive that the recuperating alcoholic obtain sufficient amounts of these vitamins daily.

It may be a good idea to take a high-potency B complex tablet once or twice a day. Be sure the tablet contains all eleven of the B vitamins. In addition to this, it may be wise to supplement the diet with extra amounts of the single B vitamins mentioned. (Try taking these vitamins after meals and not before bed.)

Among the best food sources of the B complex vitamins are liver and other organ meats, and all the muscle meats, along with wheat germ and brewer's yeast. Folic acid is also abundant in green leafy vegetables.

Vitamin C

Vitamin C, like the B complex, is unable to be stored in the body for any appreciable time. It must be regularly ingested. Most nutritional programs for alcoholic rehabilitation use large doses of this important vitamin.

It has already been noted that alcohol (ethanol) is toxic to the body. It should be added that the ingestion of alcohol seems to trigger the production of an even more toxic substance: acetaldehyde. Acetaldehyde is found in increased amounts in persons who drink large amounts of alcohol. (It is also a toxic component of tobacco smoke.) Acetaldehyde has been implicated in alcoholic heart disease, alcoholic degeneration of the brain, and addiction to alcohol.

Doctor Herbert Sprince and others at the United States Veterans Administration and Jefferson Medical College have found that the toxicity of acetaldehyde is controlled to a considerable extent by a large intake of vitamin C, and that the beneficial effect is increased by taking vitamin B1 along with it.

What is a large amount of vitamin C? According to

Nobel Prize-winner Doctor Linus Pauling: *The optimum intake without a doubt is different for different human beings . . . but probably for most of them lies in the range between 1 gram per day and 5 grams per day.* He goes on to say that some may need 10 grams (10,000 milligrams) per day.

We must remember that the alcoholic has abused his body for years. There is much rebuilding to be done. We can in no way think of the alcoholic's nutritional needs as normal.

Minerals

In addition to the minerals present in the multiple vitamin-mineral supplement which should be taken daily, it may be a good idea to add a separate multiple mineral complex. Virtually all investigators note the decreased amounts of minerals in the alcoholic. These minerals must be replaced if health is to be restored and maintained.

In addition, it might be prudent to add some extra amounts of magnesium and zinc, both of which are quickly depleted in alcoholism.

Other Helpers

There is no question that excessive consumption of alcohol is the most common cause of all categories of liver disease. Liver cells are damaged by what many would consider light drinking. Good health is not possible until the liver is in proper working order. And since the liver furnishes the brain cells with glucose and protects them from accumulating toxins, we help the brain when we help the liver.

There is a specific group of nutrients that can aid in

moving the fat out of the liver—in effect, detoxify the liver. These are referred to as "lipotropics" and are sold in tablet form. They are a combination of one or more B complex vitamins (*choline, inositol,* and sometimes *B12),* the amino acid *methionine,* and sometimes *betaine.* Since the liver has been abused such a long time, it could be wise indeed to add this special supplement to round out a complete nutritional program.

Another special aid in the treatment of alcoholism is glutamine—an amino acid constituent of protein. In the studies on rats referred to earlier in this chapter, those on poor diets consistently chose alcohol as their beverage. In a similar experiment, when rats were given glutamine, they cut their alcohol consumption by forty percent! According to Dr. Roger J. Williams: *Glutamine has helped hundreds of alcoholics.* However, he goes on to say that it does not always work like magic in a dependable fashion because we are all unique in the details of our metabolism.

Glutamine is a nutrient, not a drug, and Dr. Williams believes that *every* concerned person should give it a try. It is safe even in large amounts. Dr. Williams suggests about two grams per day. Half a gram one hour before meals and before retiring seem to bring the best results. Glutamine is tasteless and is available as tablets, capsules, and powder.

Glutamine, says Williams, *is worth trying when alcohol consumption threatens to become a problem. For many, it curbs the unhealthy desire to drink. It should be used as long as it appears to be effective.*

A Word of Caution

People manifesting alcoholism need good nutrition. The better the food and supplements the more quickly and permanently will be the response. In addition to eating only the finest foods, it should be noted that there is evidence that caffeine, nicotine, and chocolate impair recovery from alcoholism. Since none of these is a health-builder, they will eventually have to be dropped if we are to express our rightful good health.

However, giving up these things while trying to refrain from alcohol might prove to be too burdensome in the beginning. As our health improves, we will not want these subversive elements in our lives, and giving them up then will be easier.

Move We Must

No matter how nutritious the foods we eat, if the nutrients from them fail to reach the cells we will be poorly nourished. Circulation is the only way nutrients can reach cells. The simple fact is that exercise improves circulation! Without exercise the whole system stagnates. It's very clear that our bodies were designed to move, and move they must if they are to be kept in fine running order. Exercise is essential for the health of every part of the body. In order for it to be most effective, it must be done regularly.

Choose an exercise that appeals to you—one you will want to do daily. Walking is always a good choice. A long, brisk walk in the fresh air is a wonderful way to improve ourselves. Also good are swimming, cycling, golf, square dancing, yoga, and many others. Exercise is the best means we have of improving the circulation of blood, which in turn brings oxygen and other nutrients to the brain. Regular exercise means regular improvement.

"Can I Drink Again?"

Alcoholism can be cured, of that there is no doubt. To think otherwise is to believe that there is such a thing as an "incurable" disease. The reason that alcoholism can be cured is that alcoholics are "made," not "born." What is made can just as easily be unmade. In God's realm there are no such things as "alcoholics"; there are only perfect expressions of Him. If we are to be perfect we must bring that which is in God's realm into our realm.

Does this mean that a recovered alcoholic who prays, affirms health, practices good nutrition and exercises regularly can go back to drinking alcohol moderately? *Certainly not!* Alcohol is toxic to human tissues. Why would anyone want to pollute his sacred body temple—even moderately! Would we ever think that it is okay to "steal" moderately or "hate" moderately or "hurt someone" moderately? No! We know the laws of spiritual and physical health and we must follow these laws if we are to be perfect as our Father in heaven is perfect. We don't pray by asking God to change *His* laws to suit us. We pray to change ourselves so that *we* may suit God's laws.

If alcohol has been a problem in someone's life and he has overcome that problem, why would he want it in his life again? An addictive smoker who finally quits smoking would never consider smoking "moderately." If he did that he would still be a smoker because he would still have a smoker's consciousness. An overweight person who has just completed a diet and has reached his target weight may be slim now but, if he "craves" more food and "misses" his rich desserts, he is really an overweight person temporarily in a slim body because he still has an "overweight" consciousness, and until that consciousness changes he will always find a way to gain the extra weight back.

An alcoholic is cured not when he can drink moderately but when alcohol is out of his life so completely that he would never even consider drinking at all!

The Good News

If you are manifesting alcoholism now (and in your heart you know if you are), you may feel that you can never reach the point where you won't miss alcohol—but be assured that it is possible. It will happen when you realize that you are not weak or inferior or different but that you have just temporarily lost sight of the fact that you are the most magnificent creation in the entire universe. You are important to that universe, for without you creation would not be complete! You have been given dominion over all that is on the Earth. Nothing on Earth has been given dominion over you—certainly not the distilled spirits of some grain! You are a part of God and loved totally by that God who is yearning to help you but cannot do so until you turn again toward Him. God asks only one thing of each of us: that we keep His commandments—His laws. As long as we disobey the laws of Spirit, soul, or body we cannot hope to fulfill the divine mission programmed into each cell of our bodies—that of wholeness, health, and life.

Let us begin the journey back into life. Let us align ourselves again with our Creator by allowing the life force within us to express the miracle of life and wholeness. Let us begin obeying the laws of nutrition and exercise. Let us reprogram our thoughts to those of wholeness and health. Let us see ourselves as perfect expressions of a perfect Creator. Let us see it and let us believe it, for it is true!

Designs for Better Digestion

The human digestive tract is the most important highway in the world. Along it pass all the goods—the raw materials—needed for the construction of the body temple. It is the route on which travel the essential nutrients whose job it is to nourish the life force residing in our cells. Like any highway, the digestive tract must be kept open to the free flow of traffic—uncongested and unimpeded.

The stomach and small intestines are two of the organs that digest and assimilate our food. If they are not functioning properly, the vital nutrients do not get to the cells and our health suffers—the life force is deprived. When we are disobeying one or more of the many divine laws of life (be they spiritual or physical), the digestion is often one of the first voices of complaint to be heard. When the stomach speaks to us, we should listen to it, for the body is trying to tell us something.

Victor Hugo in "Les Miserables" said: *Indigestion is charged by God with enforcing morality on your stomach.* It is the life force's means of reprimanding us for having slipped somewhere along the way in our obligations to the God-ordained laws by which we were designed to live.

Stomach Is Wisdom Center

It is interesting and significant to observe that the stomach is the physical center of the judgment or wisdom faculty in the human body. This faculty is the ability we possess to reflect upon ideas with discernment, handling them in the proper way. The wisdom center in the body is directly related to good assimilation, as Charles Fillmore points out in *The Twelve Powers of Man: Every bit of food that we take into our stomachs must be intelligently and chemically treated at this center before it can be distributed to the many members waiting for this center's wise judgment to supply them with materials. . . .*

The inimitable life force in its grand omniscience knows exactly what to do with the raw materials provided it. It also knows how to heal and realign our beings so that we can express the perfection that lies ever waiting to come forth. It asks only for the proper nourishment—spiritual and physical—to help it go about its wonderful work. Once we have met our obligations—that is, provided this nourishment—we can step aside and let the life force take over. And one thing on which we can always rely is the absolute reliability of God. He can always be counted upon to do His share.

It is up to us to hold in our minds the true picture of ourselves. We must see the digestion process as being perfect, realizing that the thoughts we hold in our minds must produce their counterparts in the body. The physical body is like a living chalkboard on which is written the story of what is happening in our inner world. We can erase and add new expressions any time we choose, if we will change our thinking. *The body is the fruit of the mind. Do not talk about the body as being a low vibration or as material. In the study of mind action, take the body into consideration as the fruit of thought, and affirm that it is pure, holy, undefiled.* Again, Mr. Fillmore found the appropriate words.

Stress and anxiety are arch-enemies of the digestive system. The first place we feel it when we experience such emotions is in the pit of our stomachs. Stress is the largest single cause of stomach and duodenal ulcers and should be kept out of our lives as much as possible. This means that

149

we must change our attitudes about circumstances and people. These outer things will always be there, potentially stressful if we allow them to be. There is no way we can change that.

But what we can change is our inner world, our consciousness, our reactions to the outer world. In other words, we eliminate stress by eliminating the negative reactions that cause the stress. Things do not cause stress or bring stress to us. Only we can produce this insidious predator in ourselves.

We should never attempt to eat if we are feeling tense, anxious, or stressed in any way. The stomach will be in a "knot," the digestive juices being unable to flow properly. The result will probably be a feeling of indigestion or at least an improper assimilation of the nutrients for which the body temple has been waiting.

A good way to place the body and soul into peaceful states, receptive to the nourishment they are about to receive, is to say grace before eating. The practice of becoming still and blessing the food gives us the chance to become calm and centered. It moves us into the consciousness of awareness of the life force within us and of that life force's requirements of the finest nutrients. It helps us appreciate all the miraculous processess which are about to transpire between the time we take the first bite and the moment of jubilee when the life-giving nutrients actually are delivered to the cells.

The habit of saying grace can do much to keep us aware of who we are, as well as prepare the way for proper and peaceful digestion.

In her book *You Can Be Healed,* Clara Palmer suggests several spiritual attitudes that can prove to be excellent digestive aids: *Love is a great solvent, cheer a wonderful digestant, faith a perfect aid to assimilation. When love*

*sends its cheering message of faith into your organism, the
nerves controlling your stomach are immediately quickened
and the process of digestion is carried on speedily and in
order.*

If we are experiencing digestive problems, we can
begin to reverse them during our times of meditation.
During these daily periods of contact with our inner world,
we can actually speak (silently or audibly) to the stomach,
instructing it to do its work according to its divine design.
This is the technique Myrtle Fillmore used in her own body
healing: *It flashed upon me that I might talk to the life in
every part of my body and have it do just what I wanted. I
began to teach my body and got marvelous results.*

Digestive Devastators

In addition to stress, anxiety, and fear, there are other
devastators of the digestive system. Drugs found in coffee
act on the stomach and nervous system to increase the
stomach acid pepsin. (This substance has a lot to do with
activating ulcers.) Drugs, including aspirin, can cause
nausea and vomiting. In fact, aspirin can cause small
chemical burns in the lining of the stomach. (For this
reason, it is always wise to take aspirin or similar products
with food or milk and not on an empty stomach.) Alcohol is
another stomach "devastator." And spices, fatty foods,
fried foods, foods containing or derived from chocolate,
sugar, junk foods, and even overweight all take their toll on
digestion. They should all be scrupulously avoided.

Cooperation with the life force means being a sentinel
to every food and beverage that goes into the stomach. *The
most common cause* [of digestive problems] *is improper
eating. The cure is simple — correct your living habits. Your
stomach is a pretty tough organ and if you treat it right it will*

treat you right and (even after years of neglect) correction of your bad habits will usually result in a rapid and complete recovery. These lines appeared in the newsletter "Executive Health," which then went on to discuss the importance of good diet in the prevention and overcoming of stomach problems.

Our eating patterns must be analogous to our spiritual affirmations and denials. We must deny the junk foods, eliminating them from our lives forever. And we know that when we remove something, a vacuum is created that must be filled. In this case, we fill it with the proper life-giving foods, which are affirmations of health and perfection.

Protein is the first affirmation. Eggs, milk and milk products, cheeses, lean meat, fish, and poultry are the sources of top-grade protein the life force employs in building the body temple.

The second affirmation is carbohydrates. Constructive carbohydrates are the vital fuel of the body. These are fresh fruits, fresh vegetables, whole grains (including whole-grain breads).

The third affirmation is unsaturated fatty acids—oils. Although fats and oils might temporarily be a problem for your digestion, you do need at least a small amount of good oil in the diet each day. Margarine need not be used as it is not basically a good food. Instead, use Better Butter. You may also use a cold-pressed oil such as safflower, corn, sunflower, sesame, or soy on your vegetables, toast, and/or salads. Or, if you are using a blended protein drink, the oil can be put into that. If you have trouble digesting fats, you may want to use only small amounts of these oils at this time. Or you may not want to use any at all. However, as your digestion normalizes, you will be able to add these fine foods to your diet.

Nuts and seeds, in addition to being very healthful

snacks, are also good sources of high-quality oil in the diet. Eat them raw and unsalted. If they upset your stomach, they are not for you at this point.

Small Meals Are Big Helps

A very good method of eating for someone working to correct digestion (or for anyone interested in maximizing the efficiency of the body temple) is that of several small meals a day rather than the usual three (at least one of which is usually too large!). The stomach does not like to be overloaded. Eating frequent small meals can be an effective aid in helping the digestive system to properly process and absorb the precious nutrients.

If you decide to adopt this way of eating, make sure that each small meal contains a source of top-grade protein as well as some form of constructive carbohydrates. You might want to eat frequently by using a blended nutritious drink, which can easily be carried to work or taken in the car when you go shopping. If you decide on such a drink and are going to use a protein powder, use one made of milk and eggs rather than soy. It may be easier to digest. Here is a sample recipe that will provide the equivalent of one meal. It can be doubled or multiplied to provide the number of servings you desire:

6-8 ounces of non-fat milk or papaya juice
1 or 2 raw eggs (or yolks only)
¼ teaspoonful of a good vegetable oil
small portion of a fresh fruit
1 or 2 teaspoonsful of protein powder (If papaya juice
    is used instead of milk, use 1 tablespoonful of
    protein powder.)

You can experiment and vary the amounts and ingredients to suit your taste and needs. Essentially, however, a drink

153

such as this—sipped slowly throughout the day—will be a great boon to the overworked stomach. The key to its effectiveness is to drink it in only small amounts at a time. This is important!

There are several foods and supplements that are very helpful, soothing, and healing to the digestive tract. Aloe vera juice (1-2 teaspoonsful in about 1-2 ounces of warm water) taken right before meals is an excellent idea. Foennugreek tea and slippery elm tea are beneficial herbal beverages that soothe these membranes. Chlorophyll capsules are healing to the stomach and intestinal tissue, and acidophilus (liquid or capsules) is helpful to the colon.

Digestive enzymes are wonderful metabolic aids, not only to those with digestive problems but to anyone who wants to be certain his nutrients are being properly broken down and assimilated. There are many varieties of digestive enzymes on the market, and it is often a matter of trial and error before the appropriate one for each individual can be determined. What works for one person may do nothing at all for the next.

There are some general guidelines, however. Papaya tablets are mild and can be used as an occasional digestive aid in lieu of antacids and bicarbonate of soda, which do *not* correct the primary problem. Papaya is not effective, however, as a regular dietary supplement in helping in the assimilation of food.

Hydrochloric acid (HCl) tablets can be quite effective in the case of the bloating and uneasiness that immediately follow a meal. They should be taken just prior to the meal but must *never* be used by people who have stomach or duodenal ulcers.

Pancreatin is an excellent aid to the digestion. There are many products available that contain it either alone or combined with oxbile (which helps us digest fats and oils) and other enzymes.

Some people prefer a multiple digestive enzyme tablet that might contain several digestants, such as pancreatin, oxbile, hydrochloric acid, pepsin, and papaya (papain). These are very good. Remember to be sure to avoid the ones containing HCl if you have an ulcer.

With the exception of the plain papaya tablets, these other digestive enzymes are meant to be taken regularly. The life force delights in having such help in going about its work of wonder. Digestive enzymes can turn out to be great friends. We should not hesitate to use them.

In times of digestive stress and discomfort, we can take activated charcoal capsules. These would not be taken as regular supplements in place of digestive enzymes but merely as temporary relief for gas and indigestion. One or two capsules with warm water will often do the trick. This can be repeated every half hour if necessary. (Activated charcoal capsules are often excellent for relieving a baby's colic. The contents of ½ - 1 capsule can be emptied into warm water or warm water with a small amount of sugarless papaya syrup and put into the baby's bottle. Check with your pediatrician.)

Vitamins and Minerals for Good Digestion

There are certain vitamin and mineral supplements that we must consider. A complete multiple vitamin-mineral formula (with 10,000 or more IU's of vitamin A and the complete B complex) is a good place to start. Additional supplements of complete B complex would be even better. Extra amounts of vitamin C are necessary, but if the usual ascorbic acid form is too acid, there are other forms of vitamin C that can be taken, such as calcium ascorbate and sodium ascorbate. The calcium ascorbate would be better for those who are restricted in sodium intake.

Plenty of calcium, perhaps in the more easily absorbed form of liquid capsules, is needed to strengthen the digestive tract. It is especially helpful to people with diverticular problems, which will usually respond to a good health program as outlined here. Along with plenty of protein, many physicians feel that these people must have adequate amounts of fiber (bulk) in their diets. Fresh fruits and vegetables and whole grains—and raw bran, if necessary—provide these.

And don't forget adequate, *regular* exercise. Regular body movement is essential for regular body improvement. But be sure to do your exercises far enough away from mealtime. Very strenuous exercises should be completed at least one hour before eating or begun two hours after eating. This is important because during strenuous exercising the blood normally reserved for the organs of digestion is sent instead to the skeletal muscles. This virtually stops digestion. (Stress can have the same effect. That is why it is never wise to eat while very worried, angry, or otherwise emotionally distraught.) Less strenuous exercises can be done closer to mealtime.

All tissues, organs, and systems (including the digestive system) benefit when exercise is done. And remember, exercise *regularly*. Make it a habit you can't do without.

We must be aware of the fact that nourishing the life force does not mean simply eating the right foods, taking the right amounts of supplements, and exercising. This is only the beginning. Once these foods are introduced into the body, the divine intelligence within us begins its mighty work, silently, skillfully, without our conscious awareness. Miniature chemical factories are working at full production capacity to process the food, absorb the nutrients, and deliver them to the waiting cells, which in turn will use them to produce more life for our bodies.

The work of digestion and assimilation is phenomenal. We must never forget the magnitude of this work, nourishing is not only with our foods but also with our thoughts and aspirations toward oneness with our Creator. Therein lies the key to good digestion. When our delight is in the law of the Lord of our being and all effort is directed to Him who created us, we rise up in health and wholeness, functioning perfectly as we heed the laws He gave us. *I will praise thee, O Lord, with my whole heart; I will show forth all thy marvelous works.* And what—truly what—could be more marvelous work than a radiant and perfect human being?

"Nay, Nay" to Constipation

Have you ever stopped to think of what a terrible predicament we would be in without the power of renunciation (or elimination)? Why, we would be in a real mess! Just imagine not being able to release what you do not want.

This ability to release or relinquish the harmful and the unnecessary from our lives is so basic to our existence that it was incorporated into us as one of the twelve powers, one of the twelve divine ideas with which God endowed us. And our minds thus have the faculty (or ability) to use these powers to develop into the full Christ consciousness for which we were designed.

What a marvelous and ingenious idea it was on the part of the divine Creator to provide us with the faculty of letting go of our mistakes. The ability to say no enables us to release or deny anything we do not want in our lives. It was Jesus who referred to this "yea, yea; nay, nay" faculty, meaning our ability to affirm or deny something. And when we deny something, we are eliminating or renouncing it from our being, aren't we? In fact, sometimes we can become impacted with too many affirmations and we find that a strong no—a strong denial—is just what we need to eliminate them and clean house, so to speak.

We must always release the old in order to make room for the new. We can put just so much into our minds and bodies before they become saturated. So, if we want to grow and move forward, we are going to have to let go of the old. This is true of the mind and it is true of the body.

Wouldn't we be in a sad state of affairs if, after breathing in the oxygen-rich, life-giving air, we could not release the old, stale, carbon dioxide from our lungs? Wouldn't it be dreadful if, after the food taken into the body had served its purpose, the body had no means of eliminating the waste so that there would be room for new life-giving substances? We can think of endless examples of the necessity for release of the old, in our bodies, our minds, and in the universe around us. The Truth is that all life is a constant flow of giving and receiving, taking in and letting go. Thus, elimination is as fundamental as life itself because without it there would be no life.

Become aware of the process of renunciation at work in your world—both mental and physical renunciation. For every physical expression there exists a corresponding one in our realm of ideas. If we didn't have the power to reject and renunciate unwanted, undesirable, no longer useful ideas, beliefs, and attitudes from our consciousness, we would never develop to our full potential. *It is possible to overload the mind as one overloads the stomach. Thoughts must be digested in a manner similar to the way in which food is digested. An eagerness to gain knowledge without proper digestion and assimilation ends in mental congestion. The mind, like the bowels, should be open and free.* Charles Fillmore perceived the clear parallel between the mental and the physical. And so can we. There exists, after all, the unity of all life. Everything is related.

Anything that exists in our lives is there because we sustain the idea of it in our own minds. When we can eliminate the idea, we will eliminate the cause and, consequently, eliminate the thing itself, whatever it might be. For this reason it can simplify matters if we carefully watch everything that goes into the body or into the mind in the first place!

159

Gripping Mental Hold

It is interesting to observe what particular personality traits seem to be common among people who have trouble with their elimination. Charles Fillmore and several other metaphysicians have pointed out that almost all slowing down of the body's function of elimination is a result of the "I can't" state of mind.

Perhaps even more significant is the belief on the part of metaphysicians that these people tend to exert a gripping mental hold on their possessions. Deliberately and willfully holding on to their possessions (which can be in the form of material things and money as well as people in their lives) causes a constriction in the intestines because these organs were designed to release and let go of substance, keeping the flow open. Any willful holding on to people or possessions blocks that flow.

Charles Fillmore wrote in *The Twelve Powers of Man: The nerve center from which the eliminative function directs the emptying of the intestines is located deep in the lower bowels. This center is very sensitive to thoughts about substance and all materiality. A gripping mental hold on material things will cause constipation. A relaxation of the mind and a loosening of the grip on material possessions will bring about freedom in bowel action.* Mr. Fillmore addressed himself to this problem on several occasions, during which he stated that constipation was a common complaint of those who are *financially grasping.* This type of attitude causes the organs of elimination to *become fixed and almost immovable.*

Catherine Ponder suggests that by releasing the past we can aid our organs of elimination. But she too agrees with Mr. Fillmore that possessiveness is the cause of many cases of constipation: *It is the people who are holding on tightly and possessively to that which is no longer for their highest good that suffer most from physical ailments in the organs of elimination. . . . Possessiveness, which is one of the worst forms of bondage causing all kinds of health, financial, and human relations problems, if often reflected in the organs of elimination as disease.*

Some of these metaphysical ideas can perhaps be of help in understanding the cause of this common complaint. As always, we must go within and work with our own consciousness, for that is where all answers lie. By getting our spiritual house in order, we open the channels for all good to flow through us.

There are also the necessary physical laws to which the body temple must conform if it is to have proper elimination. When Charles Fillmore said: *God created the idea of the body as a self-perpetuating, self-renewing organism, which man reconstructs into his personal body,* he was recognizing that we were designed to operate according to these laws.

Our divine tissues can easily become littered and clogged with debris and poisonous wastes if we do not have proper elimination. It is extremely important that this renunciating faculty of our body temples remains strong and yet relaxed. Proper nutrition and exercise are essential factors in establishing and maintaining healthy elimination.

When it comes to food, we always look to protein first. It is protein that builds and repairs tissue. Every meal should therefore be built around a good source of protein. Carbohydrates—the unrefined ones—are also essential to the body temple. Unrefined carbohydrates present the body with a fine source of fiber (or bulk), which is so important to good bowel function. You can obtain extra fiber by adding one or two tablespoonsful of raw, unprocessed bran to the diet. This has been helpful to countless people. Keep in mind, however, that whole grains, fresh fruits, and vegetables are excellent sources of dietary fiber. Unlike the bran, which passes through the body undigested, the whole grains, fruits, and vegetables will supply us with life-supporting minerals and natural fuel for the body temple. We need these good carbohydrates to run smoothly.

We do not need the refined carbohydrates, such as sugar and white flour and the many "foods" into which they are incorporated. These do much to clog the large intestine, becoming impacted on the walls and causing untold disharmony in the body temple. A healthy, "Nay, nay," therefore, to all junk food!

A good oil will keep any machine well-lubricated. The miracle machine—the body temple—is no different; it needs some good vegetable oil each day.

Let's consider vitamins next. In addition to a complete multiple vitamin supplement, a good amount of the B complex is needed to restore tone to the intestines. (A complete B complex will contain eleven B vitamins. This is important.)

High amounts of vitamin C are required in overcoming constipation. This wonder vitamin helps draw moisture into the colon and is therefore very beneficial. (In fact, too large a dose of vitamin C can result in temporary diarrhea.)

Minerals are important in effecting integrity of the intestinal tissues. Calcium is of crucial importance. If the constipation is because of a spastic, constricting colon, a calcium-magnesium supplement can have a relaxing effect on the colon. If it is because of a lack of tone on the intestinal walls (which is the more common cause), extra calcium can help to strengthen these walls. Calcium might be best utilized in the form of a liquid in a capsule. Taking several at each meal and at bedtime may be helpful.

Magnesium, in addition to its calming effect, may have

a mildly laxative action in some people and so you might want to take a magnesium tablet or two daily as well. Some good forms are magnesium gluconate, magnesium citrate, and chelated magnesium. There are others. We must all experiment to see what works best for our bodies.

There are other aids worth considering. There is lecithin, a wonderful adjunct to health. Between one and three tablespoonsful of the granules a day may be a good amount. Lecithin has the added advantage of supplying the body with good amounts of the B vitamins choline and inositol—two lipotropics that will help to keep the liver healthy. In addition to this, lecithin can help to control any excesses of cholesterol in the body.

And there are digestive enzymes. One that contains some pancreatin and oxbile, in addition to aiding digestion, can help stimulate peristalsis, the motion of the intestines that propels the waste matter along. In people with constipation of long-standing, this motion has almost disappeared and often was artificially (and harshly) induced through habitual use of laxatives. We want to get away from this and restore normal function to these vital tissues. A good digestive enzyme, such as mentioned here, can help the body regain its natural ability to eliminate regularly. Take one (or more) after each meal.

Before the good nutrition and proper supplements have done their regenerating work enough to restore normal bowel function, it is advisable to use a mild herbal laxative whenever needed to prevent a build-up of body wastes. And be sure, of course, to drink plenty of water each day. This helps to eliminate poisons and keep the bowels open.

We cannot overlook the necessity for exercise. The body temple demands it for optimum health. Good exercise can do much to help overcome constipation by bringing blood to the eliminating organs. To be beneficial, exercise must be done regularly and it must be challenging to the body. A five-minute walk every morning may be regular exercise but it certainly is not challenging. Choose an exercise that will coax your body to do more than it wants to do. Excellent exercises include long, brisk walks, golf, yoga, swimming, rope-jumping, cycling, and many more. Select a form of exercise that appeals to you and be faithful to it.

Patience and Persistence

Negative conditions in the body do not occur overnight, they develop over years of abuse and apathy. We must be patient, therefore, in expecting their disappearance. With strong and steady spiritual work there is always the possibility of "instantaneous healing." But healing takes place first in the consciousness, and often we have to wait for the body to catch up with this new state of consciousness. This can take time. But we never give up, because the law always works!

If we get right spiritually, knowing (and *acting* as if we know) who we are, we will naturally strive to follow the God-made rules for the body temple. And when we do this—when we work with the law spiritually and physically—success is inevitable.

I say "nay, nay" to that which I do not want in my life and "yea, yea" to my good.

Normal Nerves are Natural

The time of business does not with me differ from the time of prayer; and in the noise and clatter of my kitchen, while several persons are at the same time calling for different things, I possess God in as great tranquillity as if I were upon my knees at the blessed sacrament.

Perhaps you are familiar with these lines by Brother Lawrence in "The Practice of the Presence of God." Brother Lawrence, a humble lay brother in France in the 1600s, lived a simple life wholly dedicated to God. His serenity and peace—even amid *the noise and clatter* of the kitchen where he worked—are consummate examples of the kind of nerves most of us would like to have.

The nerves are the metaphysical link between mind and body and, as such, it is their work to bring harmony—oneness, unity—to all the various parts of the body. The second colossal function of the human nervous system is to act as the physical organ of the mind. The entire body is meant to carry out the commands given to it by the mind, working through the brain. The brain itself is a dynamic broadcasting system transmitting power that can actually be measured in terms of microvolts.

Every cell of the body is connected to a nerve, which in turn reports its condition to the brain almost instantaneously. What an overwhelming job the brain has! It must be in constant communication with everything that is happening in the body, and it must be constantly transmitting messages from the mind. The brain is the executive of the body and, like any executive, should operate smoothly, wisely, and commandingly.

By their very natures as coordinators of the physical body and vehicles for the mind, the brain and nervous system must be kept in perfect condition. If they are not healthy, it is our duty to restore them. When we stop to realize that the nervous system is the only means by which the mind expresses itself in this life, we can begin to see the extreme importance of sound nerves. If the nervous system is not in good order, signals get crossed, thoughts get confused, and the true Christ self has a difficult time expressing.

Beware of Labels

There are many terms given to the various manifestations of nervous system disorders. We hear such names as anxiety, phobias, repressions, depression, abnormal fear, neurotic behavior, and so on. Let us not become too interested in labeling a negative condition that we would like to see gone from our lives. (We know from the second chapter of Genesis that man was given the power to name things and that whatever he decreed a thing to be it then became. So we must be careful about putting labels on things.)

It is a fact, however, that more and more people seem to be challenged by nerve problems. We, as Truth students, are most eager to have strong nerves because we are keenly aware of their importance as vehicles for Divine Mind's working in and through us. We know we must be in command of our nerves if we are to experience the peace of God that passes all understanding.

The first place to look for help for the nerves is within ourselves. This is a dichotomy because the tissues and organ (nerves and brain) that we are seeking to help are the very same tissues and organ we must use in seeking that help! But, as always, the great Creator in His infinite wisdom has designed us so that we are capable of doing this seemingly impossible feat. We turn within, then, and slowly but with certainty we begin getting our intricate nervous system in order.

Speaking of order, why not start by working with the faculty of order itself? We can know that all things must develop and operate in their right relationship to each other. There is a divine order to our lives if we will relate properly to the divine plan. We can begin to let Divine Mind take over the order of our day as we declare: *I am divine order.* This opens the way for the natural and harmonious sequence of events to flow through our day. When we stop forcing things intellectually, we allow the divine plan to unfold orderly and smoothly. We can relax and let go.

Meditation a Must

Relaxation is tantamount to good nerves. No day must ever be too hectic or too full to prevent us from spending time in meditation. The benefits from this daily experience cannot be overestimated and will readily be proved once it becomes a habit.

We need to set apart some time each day, preferably the same time every day, in which we become still in mind and body. It is often helpful to consciously direct our thoughts to each part of the body, telling it to relax; for it is only when the physical body is quiet and undemanding that the mind is undiverted and can find peace.

We must make sure, therefore, that our bodies are totally relaxed and "out of the way." Now we can focus our thoughts on the ideas of peace, harmony, and order, which will bring rest, relaxation, and new strength to the nerves.

Charles Fillmore said: *A restful state of mind is greatly to be desired because of its constructive character. When the mind is lashed by a brainstorm the cells of the whole organism are shattered and exhaustion ensues.* The storm must be quieted so that the *stream of nerve fluid,* as Mr. Fillmore refers to it, can do its proper work. He goes on to speak of . . . *the spiritual nerve fluid that God is propelling throughout man's whole being continually, as the electromagnetic center of every physically expressed atom and cell, the very elixir of life. This wonderful stream of nerve fluid finds its way over all the many nerves in man's body, giving him the invigorating, steadying power of the Holy Spirit.*

We can envision that stream of nerve fluid during our meditation. We can see and feel it coursing through our entire beings, bringing us into intimate communion with the Holy Spirit—the Christ-life, which will bring the peacefulness and order we desire.

Exercise Can Relax

Meditation is an exercise that should be practiced faithfully if we would see good results. Physical exercise works in the same manner. And physical exercise is very beneficial in calming the nerves. If you are feeling depressed, engaging in exercise with another person (providing he is cheerful and positive) can give you a lift. Perhaps walking or cycling or playing a sport with someone may prove to be good "medicine." At any rate, physical exercise is an excellent release for tensions and stresses, and time should be provided for regular periods of such activity. Regular vigorous walking is nature's antidote for stress. Many scientists believe that the impulses generated in the spindles of the muscles during prolonged walking are essential to the optimum functioning of our central nervous system.

168

Herbert deVries, PhD, director of the Physiology of Exercise Research Lab at the University of California, states: *Not only is exercise probably as effective as any tranquilizer drug, but it is also without the potential for adverse effects.* We know that all drugs have some side effects—tranquilizer drugs included. However, the only side effect evident with exercise is increased fitness.

Dr. deVries says that the exercise does not have to be too strenuous to be effective. In fact, he finds very high levels of intensity counterproductive. His data shows that rhythmic exercises such as brisk walking, jogging, cycling, swimming, and rope skipping are among the most beneficial.

Action will absorb anxiety. Choose an exercise that suits you and do it regularly—daily, if at all possible—for at least twenty minutes each time. You will feel (and see!) the difference.

In addition to meditation and physical exercise, there are other factors that can help us to achieve genuine relaxation of the nerves. Things such as a change of environment (a vacation, if it is possible), some new and cheerful colors in the home, listening to beautiful music—all these can contribute to a new sense of peace and tranquillity.

Nutrition for Nerves

There is one more factor that has an enormous role to play in the regeneration of the nerves: solid, good nutrition. We too often regard the brain and nervous system as something apart from the physical body. We make the mistake of regarding the physical brain and the *mind* as one and the same. They are not. We must realize that the laws of nutrition apply just as much to the brain and nerve tissues as they do to the rest of the body. We must realize that we weaken the brain by eating debased, processed, denatured foods. And, conversely, we strengthen the brain and nerves by eating the proper foods, full of the nutrients that are essential to the body temple.

One of the greatest discoveries of modern science is the discovery of the inseparable relationship between the nervous system and the diet. What we have eaten is directly reflected in the quality of our nerve tissues, including those of the brain. Good food, therefore, means strong nerves. The case for optimum nutrition in dealing with nervous disorders cannot be overemphasized. Let us see what some of the modern scientists are saying on the subject.

The available evidence strongly indicates that individuals suffering from these mental disorders are deficient in or dependent upon the nutrients most of us assume are being supplied by our "well-balanced diet" and sufficient water consumption. . . . We must realize that nutrition, body chemistry, and mental disease are intimately related. That from "A Physician's Handbook on Orthomolecular Medicine," edited by Dwight Kalita and the renowned and venerable Dr. Roger J. Williams.

Elsewhere in the same textbook we read this statement by the Nobel Prize-winner Dr. Linus Pauling: *Orthomolecular psychiatry is the achievement and preservation of good mental health by the provision of the optimum molecular environment for the mind, especially the optimum concentrations of substances normally present in the human body, such as vitamins.* Dr. Pauling then adds that *there is evidence that an increased intake of some vitamins . . . is useful in treating schizophrenia, and this treatment has a sound theoretical basis.* These are impressive words from men of high esteem in the scientific community.

It has been found that tranquilizers, anti-depressants, and other drugs do not solve the problem. It is a lack of proper nutrients—not a lack of, for instance, valium—which results in mental problems. "A Physician's Handbook on Orthomolecular Medicine" discusses the various foods that can cause nervous disorders. The list includes chocolate, coffee, cola drinks, alcohol, and other junk foods, with the conclusion that *medications only suppress manifestations while the disease continues and leads to irreversible changes.*

There are many other references to the importance of proper nutrition and to the unsatisfactory results of drugs. This from "Orthomolecular Nutrition" by Hoffer and Walker making reference to certain drugs is a good example: *These are useful drug molecules that do something to restore a more normal brain metabolism, but they are not naturally present in the body or the brain. They are unnatural substances which require an unnatural body and brain reaction.* In other words, nutrition and not drugs is an integral part of the composition of the body temple.

What kind of nutrition will help the brain and nervous system? Good amounts of protein are necessary. (See chapter two, page 17, for a list.) We must be sure that our breakfast includes some good protein. This is extremely important if we want the nerves to respond well for the remainder of the day. It has been established that many "nervous disorders" are actually caused by hypoglycemia (low blood sugar). This is all the more reason to be sure of getting a high-protein breakfast.

Some constructive carbohydrates should be eaten at every meal. By eliminating the destructive carbohydrates—all the junk foods that are everywhere present—and eating instead fresh fruits, fresh vegetables, and whole grains (including whole grain breads), we will go a long way in restoring balance and harmony to our ingenious nervous system. These carbohydrates are the only ones that contain the life force in abundance.

We must not forget to include some good oil in our diet too.

The Case for Supplements

So much wonderful work has been done with vitamin supplementation. Anyone seeking to perfect his nerves will undoubtedly want to investigate the possibilities of high-potency B complex (all eleven B vitamins) and large amounts of vitamin C (anywhere between 1,000 and 10,000 milligrams!). Since the B complex and vitamin C are regarded as the "stress" vitamins, they should be included in any nerve regenerating program.

In addition to the complete B complex, certain of the individual B vitamins can be helpful. Niacinamide can be taken separately in higher potencies (300 milligrams daily or more) and so can pantothenic acid. The textbook "Modern Nutrition in Health and Disease" makes this statement: *Pantothenic acid has been reported to improve the ability of* well-nourished *subjects to withstand stress.* (Emphasis added.) And the emphasis was added because it must be remembered that good health starts with a good diet. Once the proper foods are eaten, then—and only then—can we expect to obtain maximum results from our supplements.

Minerals too can be useful in strengthening the nerves. Calcium in particular is essential. Some extra magnesium is very soothing also. Begin with small amounts and see how you respond. All these are general suggestions. You are the only one who can ultimately decide what and how much of something to take. But we should not be afraid of vitamin and mineral supplements. Man was given the intelligence by God to explore new and better ways of caring for the body temple.

172

Two Special Helps

If you are eating good foods and refraining from the bad ones, and if you are taking B complex, vitamin C, niacinamide, and pantothenic acid along with a good, high-potency multiple vitamin-mineral supplement, there are two more adjuncts to your nutrition plan that might interest you. The first is lecithin.

Lecithin is necessary for good brain and nerve function. It is found in our nerve tissue. We can take lecithin (pronounced less-ah-thin) in granular form on our cereals, salads, soups, and in our blender drinks. It is a wonderful food which helps the nerves. We might try taking one or more tablespoonsful each day for maximum effect. (It is also available in oil and capsule forms, neither of which is as potent or economical as the granules.)

The second special item is glutamic acid. This is one of the amino acids found in protein and can be purchased separately as a tablet. Glutamic acid is very necessary to the brain, helping the memory and providing the raw material for some of the important chemical processes which take place in the brain. It is available in both tablet and powder form.

God First

Before this chapter is concluded, it might be wise to go back to one point. Meditation is of primary importance in establishing good mental health. While the benefits of good nutrition must not be minimized, it is important to remember that without our quiet time in "the silence" each day, we will probably not have complete success. Becoming relaxed in mind and body will do wonders for the nerves. By going within and seeking first the kingdom of God " . . . *all these*

173

things shall be yours as well." (Matt. 6:33) When we put God first, *all* good will follow—including good nerves.

Nasal Passages—Open Sesame!

If we can judge by the content of the television commercials wedged between segments of our favorite shows, sinus trouble, allergies, and colds are big business! "This is the season for head colds," we are admonished. Or, "The hay fever season is once again upon us." Or, "My sinuses are acting up."

We are led to believe that a change in temperature or the blossoming of a certain flower or some fluctuation of the weather spell doom to the nasal passages. Often those television commercials do such a good job of selling that we find ourselves expecting exactly what they are describing. And of course that is exactly what we get.

This, however, should not be. No belief in any allergy or physical imperfection must ever deprive us of the beauty and wonder of God's creation. No heat or cold, no mountains or oceans, no moisture or dryness, no flowers or trees can affect our plan for perfection when we put God first. In reality, the life force within us is the Spirit of God, which is wholeness. It cannot be affected by climatic conditions. How could it?

It is important that we are aware of this Truth and come to *really* believe it. This is the first step in the righting of any condition in the body. We must never forget our basic principle of the totality of being: Spirit, soul, and body. And we begin with the realm of the Spirit, attuning ourselves to our oneness with the Father. With this idea firmly established in our subconscious minds, we then can reach out to other aspects of our healing.

Metaphysically, we can check out ourselves for elements in our consciousness that might be contributing to discomforts of this nature. Sinus problems, for instance, can be caused by the effects of congested ideas and old resentments. Allergies can represent sensitivities to outer things—people, situations, and such. It might be that we are reacting too much to others and not "minding our own spiritual business," as Vera Dawson Tait often remarked. If this is the case, allergies can quickly disappear when we begin to see God in everyone.

Some meditative searching will soon reveal to us the metaphysical aspects of any nasal congestion. And once they are revealed, we can take steps to correct them through our prayer work and right thinking.

The nasal passages should always be clear so that we can freely draw in the very breath of God. Clara Palmer, in her book *You Can Be Healed,* refers to the nasal passages as the *gateway of life,* and she uses these words: *Every breath you draw betokens your eternal alliance with life.* We must appreciate the nose and realize that we use it to draw pure substance of Spirit into our bodies.

The Power of Song

Another area with which we can work is that of the power faculty—the power center located in the throat at the base of the tongue. This is one of the twelve powers of which Charles Fillmore spoke. The spoken word, authoritatively delivered, is recorded in the body tissues. We can speak powerful words of Truth to our cells. But we can go even further than speaking the word—we can *sing* it!

Singing is therapeutic because it is a release for pain. It buoys our spirits and lightens our souls. It does even more than that, however: the vibrations of the voice can actually change the chemistry of the cells and serve to reverberate through the sinus cavities, breaking up old crystallized conditions—mental and physical.

So, singing is good exercise. And, speaking of exercise, there are other things you can do. It has been found that any good physical exercise can help open the nasal passages. It should not be too strenuous at this time, but should be active enough to provide some good relief.

Walking is a good exercise. A brisk walk in the fresh air does wonders for the entire body. There are many other good exercises, such as swimming, boating, square dancing, hiking, bowling, yoga, horseback riding, etc. Choose the one that is best for you and do it regularly. You will like the results.

The Manifest Substance

Let us move into the area of nutrition now and see what can be done by following the physical laws God gave us for maintaining our priceless body temples. Myrtle Fillmore fully appreciated the necessity of following these laws when she wrote: *We must agree to think health, and to bless the body, and to express that which causes all the functions of the organism to work perfectly. But there is the physical side of health also. Spirit must have substance through which to manifest! You must provide the manifest substance and life elements in proper food, and drink, and sunshine, and air. Without these, Spirit would have no vehicle.* How true, how true!

There are specific manifest substances and life elements which, when taken into the body, can be utilized for the purpose of building health and eliminating any sinus, allergy, or cold problems. Let us take a look at these nutrients.

As always, we begin by checking the protein intake. Are we eating some eggs or milk or cheese or lean meat or fish or poultry at every meal, including (and especially) breakfast? If not, this is the place to start correcting our diet. No meal is complete without a good source of protein.

Next, we need a good carbohydrate source at each meal.

We also need some good oil each day. It should be a cold-pressed oil that contains no preservatives and, therefore, must be kept refrigerated. (See chapter two, page 17, for proper sources and amounts.)

In addition to the health-building foods, certain supplements will prove very helpful to you.

A good complete multiple vitamin-mineral supplement is always good insurance. It is one of the many ways in which we can let the life force know we appreciate its ceaseless efforts on our behalf. And if you take some extra B complex, so much the better.

It is vitamin A and vitamin C, however, that stand out as extremely important to the delicate tissues of the nasal passages. Extra vitamin A can help strengthen them into the resilient tissues they were designed to be.

Vitamin C is our superstar here. If you have already discovered the great benefits of this marvelous vitamin and are taking enough of it, you may have eliminated colds from your life. If you have tried all else and are still manifesting sinus problems, colds, and/or allergies, make haste for the nearest bottle of vitamin C.

There have been several fine books written on the research done with ascorbic acid (which is a scientific name for vitamin C) among which are "Vitamin C and the Common Cold" by Dr. Linus Pauling and "The Healing Factor" by Dr. Irwin Stone. Their evidence is enough to convince almost anyone of the importance of ingesting enough of this important vitamin.

How much vitamin C to take? We can only tell you that your own body will tell you. Many scientists suggest that an adult needs 1,000 to 5,000 (some say 10,000) milligrams daily. Work up in your amounts until you see a difference in your nasal passages. (Since there is virtually no toxicity to the vitamin, high amounts are well-tolerated.) You will soon find your appropriate level and, when you do, stay with it.

Assuming that you are taking minerals, at least in your multiple supplement, there is one special mineral that should be added in greater amounts. This is calcium. We need calcium to build strength into the nasal tissues and make them less sensitive to external conditions. Try some extra calcium. The body knows instinctively how to convert it into living elements that are then incorporated into the tissues.

Gustaf Stromberg, in his splendid book "Man, Mind, and the Universe," refers to this inscrutable body wisdom: *We do not have to understand how the Superior Wisdom works. We can be satisfied with the knowledge that It does work. Now and always. And we can use it!*

Let us give the body these nutrients, therefore, and let its own *Superior Wisdom* work with them and use them as only it knows how. *I praise thee, for thou art fearful and wonderful. Wonderful are thy works! Thou knowest me right well.*

A Special Drink

It is time to mention a most effective and simple aid. If you have been obeying all of God's laws for good nutrition, there is a special drink you can make that can pop open those congested passages. But the proper foods must be eaten too, since there is no shortcut to good health. There is just no way to break a law that the Creator has ordained.

Here is the drink: Dissolve one teaspoonful of vitamin C powder or crystals plus two teaspoonsful of liquid chlorophyll (or one-half teaspoonful of the powder) in a glass of water. Sip on this over a period of several hours. When it is gone, make another batch. The object is to keep sipping until the nasal passages dry up. Each of us is a unique individual, so we each must find our own point at which the drink works. But work it will. Take note of about how much vitamin C powder it took to reach the point of effectiveness. That is *your* level and should be continued for at least another day and used again any other time the symptoms appear. It should be noted that if too much vitamin C is taken at one time, it could result in diarrhea and/or excessive amounts of intestinal gas. The liquid chlorophyll usually serves to buffer this effect, however, as well as being a purifying agent.

There are so many marvelous things available to us for use in working with the life force within us. This drink is one of those remarkable discoveries. We know you will be pleased with the results you get from it. And those nasal passages will be so grateful!

There is no reason why sinus problems, allergies and colds cannot become things of the past if we follow the divine laws set before us. This means that we become aware of our oneness with the Creator and, in so doing, we lift our consciousness to levels where we see the perfection of our being. It means we exercise this miracle machine, which is the temple of the living God. It means we select only the finest, most health-building foods, which the Spirit within can transform into healthy tissues.

We were given the ability and the potential to attain perfect health. *Man's true mission,* writes Richard Lynch in

The Secret of Health, is to be a (co-creator) with God, an interpreter of pure intelligence, a supervisor of the work of living molecules, an architect of cosmic design. All material has been furnished him; innately he holds the magic formula of perfect manifestation. It is all there within us! The magic formula is already ours. Bless your nose, bless your sinuses; they are about to become perfect.

Thank You, Father for the breath of life that fills my being and thrills my soul.

Down with Diabetes!

Joyous radiant health is the result of the right spiritual viewpoint, the daily purposeful effort to unfold the faculties and soul qualities, and the daily recognition of the body as the temple of God and the structure that Spirit and soul are building, all these prompting us to give careful attention to the needs of the system. Any weakness, sickness, inharmony, imperfection in the organism is the result of some failure to identify oneself with God, the divine Source, and understanding how to lay hold of and express one's inheritance of spiritual powers; some limitation in the soul's development of its riches; some ignorance of the body's requirements, and disregard of the divine law of life and health.

Myrtle Fillmore (the cofounder of Unity) certainly said a mouthful in that paragraph. Let us look closely at what it is telling us, because in essence it is the formula for health. Upon review, we find that three factors are necessary in order for us to manifest perfect wholeness. There is the "right *spiritual* viewpoint"; there is "*soul* unfoldment"; and there is "recognition of the *body* as the temple of God"—Spirit, soul, and body—the living trinity of a magnificent human being. Any dis-ease in the organism, therefore, is the result of the misuse of one or more of these three aspects. Perhaps we are not realizing our spiritual oneness with the universal life force; maybe we are in some way impeding the development of our souls; or it could be that we are not operating according to the physical laws that are part of the divine plan for the body temple.

We must investigate each area (Spirit, soul, and body) to ascertain where the weakness lies. What are the causes of the effect known as, for example, diabetes? Perhaps there is work to be done in all *three* of the areas. We do not know. Only you, the individual, can discover these causes for yourself through diligent and perspicacious introspection — self-examination.

Beginning with the spiritual, because all things proceed from Spirit, we work daily with our meditation and prayer to quicken our awareness that: *I and the Father are one.* Through seeking first the kingdom of God, all else falls into place along the way and we are promised: *"Then shall your light break forth like the dawn, and your healing shall spring up speedily."* (Isaiah 58:8)

Meditation also provides us with the opportunity to work on the development of our souls. What mental attitudes do we consistently repeat? What feelings and emotions do we find ourselves expressing? Are our patterns positive or negative? These are not easy questions to answer to the fullest. The only way to really discover the answers to such questions is through daily meditation. There just does not seem to be any way to get around that fact. The Truth is always within ourselves, and it is only through regular periods of silent contemplation that we begin peeling back the multitudinous layers of our minds to discover the Truth of our beings. The more one meditates, the more light is revealed.

One thought that could be taken into meditation is this: "Could it be that I am feeling a lack of the sweetness of life in my world?" Diabetes can often be explained metaphysically as a condition arising out of feelings of bitterness and resentment. The sweetness has gone out of life, so to speak, and so the body begins compensating for this by creating an internal environment in which the sweetness (sugar) is retained. It seems to be an idea worth reflecting upon during meditation.

Physiologically, diabetes is a breakdown in the body's ability to handle carbohydrates properly. In its most common form, certain cells in the pancreas do not secrete an adequate amount of insulin, and the blood sugar is therefore elevated. There are other factors involved, but this is basically what is happening in the body. More work can be done through meditation, this time by speaking to and praising the various parts of the body, such as the pancreas. Charles Fillmore taught: *Through thought you must work Truth into every part of your body temple. This is not too difficult, but it requires attention and persistence.*

Bless the pancreas and liver. Encourage them to do their wonderful work efficiently and perfectly, according to their divine design. Myrtle Fillmore and many others have achieved remarkable success through this method. You can too.

The Needs of the System

Attuning ourselves spiritually to the allness of God and meditating each day on the various aspects involved in our souls' development, there is one further step that needs to be taken. We should, as Myrtle Fillmore said: . . . *give careful attention to the needs of the system.* There are specific laws that must be observed if we are to expect and experience total health.

Physical exercise is one of the laws of the body temple. We were designed to move. It is essential then that we regularly engage in some form of good physical exercise. Walking has been described as the best all-around exercise, but it must be brisk and regular in order to be most effective.

Cycling, swimming, and yoga are good too. Whatever type of exercise you choose, do it regularly and joyfully.

James F. Toole, MD, writing in "Executive Health," makes this interesting report: *Late-onset diabetes is almost entirely reversible by exercise if you are overweight.* What he is saying is that if you are overweight and have developed diabetes in the adult years, you stand a very good chance of overcoming the disease through proper exercise. Exciting news! That seems like a good trade-off, doesn't it—some regular exercise for diabetes and your extra weight thrown in (or should we say "out") with the bargain.

Exercise is vital. What was said of the need for regular meditation holds true for physical exercise—there is simply no substitute for it.

Prayers in Action

There is no way to get around the laws of proper nutrition. If we get "right" in the other areas—spiritual, mental, and exercise—but stop short of the laws of nutrition, we cannot expect to permanently overcome diabetes (or any other physical challenge). To disregard these physical laws, which were created by God for our welfare, is to deny our prayers and affirmations for health. Our deeds—our right actions on behalf of God's laws—are our evidence to our Creator that we *really* believe that the life force dwells within the body temple. Our good works (e.g. eating properly) convince the Creator that we mean business! Without these good works, our prayers and affirmations fade into the dim mists of the forgotten past, where they are dissipated into nothing more than hollow phrases of wishful thinking, no matter *how* we had hoped our thoughts and words would in themselves have done the trick.

No, alas, it doesn't work that way. The actions of our

lives bespeak our *truest* prayers—and it is *these* which always do get answered. *"The works that I do in my Father's name, they bear witness to me."* (John 10:25)

It becomes important, therefore, to learn the laws of the body temple so that we can do the works that will fulfill those laws. We look first to protein. So much of the body is constructed of protein. It is needed for all qualitative growth and repair of the tissues. Even the hormone so directly related to sugar metabolism—insulin—is a protein. We must be sure to eat adequate amounts of this life-producing food.

Eggs, milk and milk products, cheeses, including cottage cheese, fish, poultry, and very lean meats, are the best sources of top-grade protein. As such, at least one of these fine foods should be included in each meal. Breakfast, especially, should be a nutritious meal containing a good, high-grade protein. A good breakfast is fundamental to good health. If you don't like to eat breakfast, drink it in the form of a blended protein drink. It will make a difference in the way you feel and act.

It is not necessary to eat all of the top-grade proteins. Some may not like milk, others cheese. Still others may not want to eat any flesh foods. That is fine. You can express perfect health without eating all these foods. However, it is generally best to use foods from this list to satisfy your protein requirement. If you want to shun animal foods completely, it is still possible to express good health. However, it is essential that you learn how to combine your fruits, vegetables, grains, nuts, and seeds to improve their amino acid balance and thereby render them better protein sources. Be scientific about this food combining. It is extremely important.

Most diabetics eat too little protein and too much of the wrong carbohydrates. And wrong (refined, processed) carbohydrates are a disaster in the body temple. This from "A

Physician's Handbook of Orthomolecular Medicine": *Over-eating of concentrated refined foods puts an unnatural strain on the pancreatic production of insulin, although it may take as long as twenty years to culminate in diabe-tes. . . . While sugar does provide quick energy, which may be useful in an emergency, it is like burning gasoline in a home furnace. It will burn, but it wrecks the machinery.*

Sweet Becomes "Sour"

When the proper protein food is eaten, along with the constructive carbohydrates, there will not be the craving for something sweet. In fact, in time, anything sweet and sugary will be repugnant! You can observe this in yourself. Eliminate the junk foods from your diet. No more sugar, white flour, candy, ice cream, soft drinks, diet drinks, alcohol, cookies—oh, the list is endless, isn't it? The list of the destructive carbohydrates can go on for pages, while the list of *constructive* carbohydrates—those that the body can handle and use properly as fuel—is very short. The con-structive carbohydrates—those containing the life force in abundance are: fresh fruits, fresh vegetables, and whole grains (which can include whole-grain breads if made with-out sugar).

These—and only these—are the raw materials God provided us with to be used as fuel in the body temple. The right carbohydrates give us energy and do not cause prob-lems with our sugar-metabolizing mechanisms. We must always beware of the junk foods; they are destroyers. Since there is no such thing as a neutral food, what we eat and drink is either going to help us or hurt us. *In effect, a junk diet is a disease diet, especially resulting in the so-called de-generative diseases of civilization such as heart problems, and forms of cancer, arthritis, and diabetes,* say Hofer and

Walker in "Orthomolecular Nutrition."

Our third food group is fats and oils. The inclusion of a good source of oil in the diet is part of the law. We need the unsaturated fatty acids, which such oils as safflower, sunflower, corn, sesame, soy, and others provide. The best ones are the cold-pressed varieties usually found in health food stores. One or more teaspoonsful daily will supply essential factors to the body. Part of that daily quota could be in the form of cod liver oil or wheat germ oil (in liquid or capsule form), and that would add extra benefits.

Nuts and seeds, in addition to being fine, tasty snacks, are a good source of many nutrients including oil in the diet. Eat them raw and unsalted.

Artificial sweeteners should not be used. "Not used? But how can I eat something that isn't sweetened?" you ask. Well, we have already seen that once the proper amounts of protein are eaten and the constructive carbohydrates are used, the body will no longer crave sweetened foods. In the meantime, if you need to sweeten something, you might find that you can use very tiny amounts of tupelo honey, which is not so insulin-dependent as other types of honey. *But before doing so, be sure to ask your physician!* If you feel you must resort to using the artificial sweeteners, do so with the intention of giving them up as soon as possible. They are not helpful to the body temple.

We must now consider some very important vitamins that are helpful in rehabilitating the pancreas and liver, the latter also being involved in carbohydrate metabolism. Vitamin A is needed, so we should be taking a good multiple vitamin supplement containing good amounts of vitamin A (10,000 International Units or more). Next we need good amounts of the complete B complex. (Perhaps in addition to that which you get in your multiple formula you might want to take some extra B complex tablets.) The multiple tablet should also contain some vitamin D, vitamin E, and vitamin C in addition to a supply of minerals. This multiple vitamin-mineral formula will assure at least a minimum amount of nutrients in the daily diet.

Extra amounts of vitamin C may also be helpful. Most of us do not take as much as our bodies require. We cannot make this important vitamin in our own bodies and must rely on outside sources. Supplementation of 3,000 milligrams or more daily is recommended by many scientists and clinical researchers.

We also need minerals. These too cannot be made in the body and must be obtained from outside sources. Our foods may not yield enough to supply us with the amounts necessary to overcome the stresses placed upon the body by diseases such as diabetes. It is prudent, therefore, to take at least a good multiple mineral complex. Extra calcium may be useful too.

Recently it has been determined that one of the trace minerals, chromium, is related to carbohydrate metabolism. In a paper published in the "Journal of Applied Nutrition," Volume 31, Numbers 1 and 2, 1979, Dr. M. Taher Fouad writes extensively on the research done on this subject. Here is a key statement: *It is, therefore, obvious that chromium is an essential trace element, but also participates as an important factor in restoring glucose tolerance in man where clinical signs of diabetes have been confirmed.*

The finest food sources of chromium are brewer's yeast and whole grains where, combined with other important molecules, it forms something called the glucose tolerance factor (GTF).

The human body is made up of and requires *all* the nutrients. We have been discussing only the ones that would seem to be especially needed for diabetes. There is one other supplement that often proves to be beneficial in helping to regenerate the pancreas, and that is pancreas substance and pancreatic enzymes. It has always been a maxim of the homeopathic physician that *similia similibus curantur,* "like cures like." For this reason, these items are often added to a nutritional program for diabetes. They can help restore good function to those very special cells in the islets of Langerhans which produce insulin. One or two pancreatic enzymes after each meal could prove to be advantageous.

Here has been presented a threefold approach to overcoming diabetes. We have seen how we must direct our attention to each of the three aspects—Spirit, soul, and body. As we work with the laws of all three, our health *must* improve. We can expect it. Please note this special admonition: If you are now taking insulin, it will be important to check frequently with your physician to determine your insulin requirements. As your health increases, your need for insulin will decrease. It is very important that you be monitored for this change. Do not change your intake of insulin under any circumstances, however, without your doctor's instruction to do so.

Lastly, we must always remember the true source of all healing. All means employed (medication or meditation, vitamins, or insulin) are methods by which the life force works its miraculous healing stream throughout our divine tissues. This chapter opened with a quote from Myrtle Fillmore. Let's end with one too: *The Christ presence within our own soul is the Great Physician who has wisdom and power to heal and to adjust in divine order every function of our body temple.*

Help for the Hyperactive

*Train up a child in the way he should go, and when he
is old he will not depart from it.* (Proverbs 22:6)

What an awesome responsibility we have to our children. We must provide the very best spiritual, emotional,
mental, and physical environment possible for them in
order that their souls have every advantage to develop and
move toward their true potential. At times the responsibility
may seem almost an impossible one, especially if we have a
hyperactive child in the home. Anyone who has been in the
company of such a child for more than a short time soon
realizes the frustration and irritation that can be experienced.

Hyperactivity is on the rise, our statistics tell us; and it is
not confined to childhood. This condition is becoming prevalent in adults as well. But it is not a hopeless challenge, as
many would believe. There is a way out—a way that leads
back to health and serenity and permanent well-being. The
solution lies in the observance of the laws that govern our
three-fold nature: Spirit, soul, and body. Each aspect must
be given proper attention, nurture, and love.

The time to begin is the earliest days of childhood. It
can never be too soon to care for the spiritual, mental, emotional, and physical needs of the child. Children want this.
They subconsciously crave it; and they are unable to provide it for themselves. " . . . *I am but a little child; I do not
know how to go out or come in.* " (I Kings 3:7) Too often we
ignore the needs of the young child, refusing to see him as a
unique individual soul, and thereby not providing him with

the material for development for which his soul hungers. We sometimes do not realize that these are eternal souls clothed in young bodies, and so we turn our attention from them, not recognizing that they "know." Thus we read in Lamentations 4:4: *. . . the children beg for food, but no one gives to them.* The "food" referred to here is not only physical food but can be interpreted as spiritual food in the form of guidance and understanding, which leads to their spiritual growth.

The first step in working with a hyperactive child (or adult) is that of providing an air of peace and harmony in the home. The flow of spiritual love should pervade the atmosphere as we continuously hold the image of the child as perfect and at peace.

We therefore must cease reacting to the behavior of the child (unsavory as it may appear) and begin treating him as the perfect child he is meant to be. This becomes easier to do as we are able to behold the Christ at the center of each person. And the only way we can behold the Christ in others is to first contact the Christ center in ourselves. Once we have centered ourselves, the Christ nature in the child will be evident, and we will then be able to interact with the child on a much higher plane—center to center. Without this first step, there is little hope of any permanent success.

The faith faculty of the parents is to be developed. The constant use of affirmations is very effective in helping the *parents* to develop this faith and thereby be in a good position to help the child. When the parents' faith is strong enough, they can begin to affirm the Truth for the child, gradually building peace and poise into his very tissues. Charles Fillmore described it with these words: *By affirmation the mind lays hold of living words of Truth and builds them into the body.* Simple, direct Truth statements can be spoken to the child, often with very good results. For exam-

ple, you might affirm: *You are peaceful and composed.* Or
you may want to say: *You are quiet and calm — a perfect
child of God.* Make up one that suits you and your child and
affirm it constantly.

The fact is that the spiritual and physical welfare of the
child is so much in the hands of the parents. These little
ones do not know how to care for their many needs.

If we are confronted with the situation of a hyperactive
child, let us reexamine the needs of that child and rededi-
cate ourselves to serving those needs. We must. Who else
can do it? They cannot. The responsibility, alas, is ours.

The spiritual environment has already been discussed.
We begin with that. Next we can consider the actual physical activity itself. Proper time must be set aside for disciplined play and/or sports, depending on the age of the
child. It has been said that order is the first law of the universe. All creation, including little children, functions best
when observing order. The runaway nerves of the hyperactive child can be gently coaxed back into line with *loving*
discipline. (The key word is *loving.*) In this way the physical
activity becomes a channel for the heretofore uncontrolled
energies, with the result that the child grows happier and
less tormented by his own nerves.

This regular period of disciplined physical activity can
gradually be led to include some of the more passive types
of activity. The playing of quiet games, and eventually the
listening to or reading of stories can be introduced. All this,
however, with great love and patience on the part of the
parents, who must never waver in their ability to see the
child as perfect—not perfect as they believe in perfection
from their human viewpoint, but perfect as the unfolding
individualization of the life force seeking to do the will of the
Father. There is a difference!

193

Right Foods Work Wonders

Finally, we come to the subject of the nutritional needs of the hyperactive child. Oh, what a subject this is! The result of work being done by scientists in the field of nutrition as it relates to hyperactivity is nothing short of sensational. This quote from "A Physician's Handbook of Orthomolecular Medicine" is evidence: *Control of the child's diet is an integral part of the total treatment, and failure to improve the child's nutritional status can be responsible for achieving minimal results. Greater concern must be shown for the quality of the child's inner environment in which his cells and tissues function if we are to help him attain optimal performance. The removal of offending foods from the diet of disturbed or learning disabled children can result in dramatic improvement in behavior, attention span, and concentration. . . . It has been the universal observation of these investigators who assess the child's nutritional status that they eat a diet which is richest in sugar, candy, sweets, and in foods made with sugar. The removal of these foods results in a dramatic decrease in hyperactivity.*

Could any statement be clearer? The chapter goes on to explain how parents must be made to realize that they *litter their children's bodies* by letting them have all those unnatural junk foods. These false foods should not even be brought into the home. Proper nutrition should be practiced by the parents as an example to the child, who is usually bombarded by television commercials urging him to beg Mommy to buy some trashy "food" which will devastate his divine tissues. Horrors!

So we remove, as best we can, all the sugar and artificial "foods" from the child's diet. This is imperative. Then we begin introducing wholesome, nutritious foods into his body temple. There must be plenty of protein for growth and for rebuilding the nerves. So be sure to include eggs, milk, cheese, fish, poultry, or meat—at least one of these health-builders—at each meal, and a small amount as a snack whenever the child is hungry.

The *correct* carbohydrates are important. Let's substitute fresh fruits and vegetables and whole grains (whole grain, *sugarless* bread included) for those destructive, false carbohydrates (such as cakes, cookies, candy, soft drinks, sugared breakfast cereals, and the like). The change in behavior will be noticeable. If you *must* sweeten something, use only honey, blackstrap molasses, sorghum, raw cane syrup, or pure maple syrup. Keep in mind that these foods are very concentrated so use only *very small* amounts. This is important.

Apple or Candy?

How about using natural, sugar-free juices instead of those pop drinks? How about an apple instead of a candy bar? How about a handful of raw nuts and seeds instead of potato chips? The possibilities are vast. Just remember that good, wholesome food is what the life force within those cells wants and needs—and deserves!

And of course we must see to it that the child gets adequate essential fatty acids each day. These are found most abundantly in oils such as safflower, sunflower, corn, soy, and sesame. Such good-tasting oils should be used raw. They can be put on salads, vegetables, baked potatoes, and in soups. Better Butter can be used wherever you would normally use regular butter. (See chapter two, page 24, for recipe.) Cod liver oil, although not a good-tasting oil, is also rich in essential fatty acids, and as an extra bonus, is high in vitamins A and D—both of which are needed by growing young bodies. (Cod liver oil comes flavored and also in capsule form to make it more palatable.)

Other good sources of oil are in nuts and seeds. These are wonderful foods and make marvelous snacks. They are best eaten raw and unsalted.

It is important to stay with as simple and natural a menu as possible. Processed, adulterated, prepacked, preserved food items have no place in the life of one who is seeking to properly care for the body temple. There is just no way to escape that fact. Food additives, artificial colorings, and preservatives are particularly harmful to the hyperactive and *must* be taken out of the diet.

Drs. Clyde Hawley and Robert Buckly, writing in "The Journal of Applied Nutrition" about the effects of food dyes on hyperactive children (and adults), have this to say: *Disturbed behavior in children can result from . . . a sensitivity to aniline coal tar compounds.* They go on to say: *The presence of the aniline coal tar dyes in processed foods has been found to be causally related to behavior disturbance in a significant number of hyperkinetic children.* These dyes are commonly used in many "quick energy" and prepared foods like TV dinners, soft drinks, ice cream, hot dogs, cakes, pies, and many more. In fact, the use of these dyes is so widespread that these investigators found: *. . . only one brand of vitamin drops for infants that did not contain additives obviously selected to appeal to the mother.*

Special emphasis must be placed upon a good breakfast. This meal is the key to daily nutrition. It should be built around good proteins (eggs, milk, cheese, or meats) and bolstered by a constructive carbohydrate, such as fresh fruit, whole grain cereal, or toast. The hyperactive child *must* eat a good breakfast. If he doesn't like eggs, try a hamburger patty or a "milk shake" made with milk, protein powder, ripe banana (or other fresh fruit) and honey. A raw egg or yolk can be added as can carob powder. (The carob powder will give it a chocolate look and taste.) Be inventive and make it tasty—but find *something* nutritious that he will eat. *This is critical to his recovery.* No child should ever be sent off to school without a good breakfast. Make it a rule.

Success with Supplements

In addition to correct diet, vitamin and mineral supplementation should be carefully considered. Here is another quote from "A Physician's Handbook of Orthomolecular Medicine": *There is rapidly accumulating evidence that a child's ability to learn can be improved by the use of large doses of certain vitamins, of mineral supplements, and by improvement of his general nutritional status through removal of "junk foods" from his daily diet. With orthomolecular treatment, results are frequently quick in starting and the reduction in hyperactivity often dramatic.* (The authors define orthomolecular medicine as *essentially the treatment and prevention of disease by the expert adjustment of the natural chemical constituents of our bodies. It places its reliance on these agents (vitamins, minerals, etc.) in preference to chemicals and drugs which are foreign to healthy metabolism. Nutrition . . . plays a dominant role in orthomolecular medicine.*)

Just what supplements are useful in treating hyperactivity? The complete B complex is necessary. (This is eleven B vitamins in one tablet.) Older children and adults can take *extra* niacinamide, which is one of the B vitamins.

Large amounts of vitamin C are good, as is a plentiful supply of a calcium-magnesium supplement to calm the nerves. Glutamic acid, one of the amino acids found in protein, can be purchased separately and is helpful to the brain. All these supplements can be crushed and dissolved in juice if the child is too young to swallow tablets.

If a physician who is familiar with orthomolecular medicine or a professional nutritionist who is familiar with it is available for you to work with, fine. If not, begin always with small amounts of supplements and work up from there.

The program outlined in this article can provide you with a new perspective—an open door—through which the answer to hyperactivity can come. It is a project that will take effort in both the spiritual and physical areas. But it is a project that can be utterly rewarding because the results will be that of an unfolding soul's finding rest and contentment at last within the confines of its own body temple.

High Hopes for Hypoglycemia

The miraculous human body is in many respects similar to a powerful dynamo. It converts one form of energy to another. And, like the dynamo, the body itself must be powered by some source of energy—some type of fuel. The major fuel for the human body is glucose, which is also known by the name "blood sugar."

When there is insufficient fuel in the body, we say there is "low blood sugar" or "hypoglycemia," and the body engine begins to stall. There are many people who (usually through years of faulty diets) have lost the ability to metabolize their foods, especially their carbohydrates, in a normal manner. The result is generally one of two conditions: *hypo*glycemia (low blood sugar) or *hyper*glycemia (high blood sugar, or diabetes). The two are merely opposite sides of the same coin and often manifest similar symptoms.

Diabetes was discussed in an earlier chapter. We will concern ourselves here with its opposite—hypoglycemia.

Many of us have this condition and don't know it. We feel there is something not quite right with the body temple, but we cannot seem to pin it down. We are not actually "sick," and sometimes it is not diagnosed.

"It is all in your mind," we are often told. But anyone who has ever experienced the discouraging symptoms of low blood sugar knows it is more than in the mind. Nervousness, irritability, anxiety, loss of concentration, crying spells, unidentifiable fears and apprehensions, dizziness, weakness, tiredness, shakiness, and even fainting—these and many other symptoms are familiar to the hypoglycemic, who can experience from one to several of these distressing signs.

We all experience some of these emotions at one time or another. We all have fears or nervousness occasionally in our lives. We accept them for what they are—the result of an unusual situation—and proceed to change either the situation or (even better) our reaction to the situation. After dealing with the problem, the negative emotion is no longer viable and we are able to resume our normal lives.

However, those suffering from hypoglycemia, or low blood sugar, experience many of these emotions nearly all the time! They are unable to identify the situation causing them or, if they can, they find themselves physically and emotionally incapable of dealing with it. To try to meditate and enter into communion with one's Creator while in such a state of distress is very difficult. We can best grow spiritually when the physical body is at ease and can be forgotten. If for no other reason than that of facilitating meditation and spiritual growth, the problem of low blood sugar must be overcome.

The habitual nightmares of fatigue, headaches, dizziness, weakness or other equally agonizing symptoms must be eliminated, and they *can* be. There *is* help for the hypoglycemic who falls apart at the smallest physical or emotional stress and often fears he is becoming insane.

Hypoglycemia is a too-often undiagnosed malady affecting literally millions of Americans of all ages, and it is often prominently involved in such diverse problems as hyperactivity, schizophrenia, depression, suicide, drug abuse, alcoholism, learning disabilities, epilepsy, and a plethora of other physical and emotional disorders. Just what is hypoglycemia and how can it be treated? Let's take a look.

God Dwells in Cells

Any discussion of hypoglycemia, or indeed of any problem affecting our bodies, must *begin* with the realization that our bodies are made up of a community of billions upon billions of tiny, hardworking cells. Life begins on the cellular level. But a crucial point to be made is that within each of these hardworking cells of our bodies there exists a universal life force which seeks only wholeness, health, and life. It knows nothing about disease; it knows nothing about decay; and it knows nothing about death. It knows only life and seeks only life. And it does so because it must follow a divine design within the cell. This design is a blueprint for perfection. Charles Fillmore said: . . . *Health is fundamental in Being and . . . is [our] divine birthright. . . . Health is the normal condition of man and of all creation.*

The fact that we may not be manifesting that health or perfection at the present time is not the fault of the design, for the design is perfect; it is made by the master architect in His own image and likeness. No, if the structure is faulty, it is the fault of the builder. If our bodies show weaknesses or frailties, then it is we, the builders, who have inhibited the full expression of its grandeur. We have done this by perverting the expression of the life force with our thoughts of limitation. James Allen put it beautifully in his poem "As a Man Thinketh":

Mind is the Master-power that moulds and makes,
And Man is Mind, and evermore he takes
The Tool of thought, and, shaping what he wills,
Brings forth a thousand joys, a thousand ills;
He thinks in secret, and it comes to pass:
Environment is but his looking-glass.

So we must begin our quest toward health and wholeness by first turning our thoughts toward God; for, in all journeys, in all endeavors, in all quests—God first! If we put God first in our lives and seek His kingdom, then in the course of our seeking all good will come to us. " . . . *seek his kingdom, and these things shall be yours as well.*" (Luke 12:31)

Next, let us put all thoughts of past sicknesses and disorders where they belong—in the past—and begin living in the now! Let us deny that which is false about us—namely, that it is somehow "our nature" to be sick. Let us affirm that which we know is true—namely, that in potential *we are perfect* and that only *we* can allow that perfection to unfold, and that today—at this very moment—we will begin to do so! We will begin to allow that life force within us to express our full potential, and it will do so because today—at this very moment—we will begin seeking first the kingdom of God.

In our seeking, let us not forget to obey all God's laws, for existing on the physical plane means obeying physical laws, no matter how much we may deny their existence. As Charles Fillmore said: *All sane persons acknowledge the necessity of observing the laws of health in their daily lives.* Let us be sure to realize that we must function within the boundaries of our present state of consciousness. If in our present state of consciousness we must eat food in order to live, then let's not eat harmful food and expect to be healthy, no matter how strongly we affirm that it will not hurt us. When we plant tomato seeds, we cannot harvest corn. When we eat lifeless foods, we cannot harvest health. Remember, the life force resides in the foods that God created.

It has already been mentioned that we are a community of cells. These cells do not exist as isolated entities but are joined together to form a most amazing "machine"—the human body. And what a marvelous machine it is to behold. But, as already stated, in order for this machine to run properly, the cells need a very specific kind of fuel, and that fuel is glucose or blood sugar. The more efficiently this glucose is distributed to the cells, especially the cells of the brain, the smoother the operation of the body. It is when the distribution system breaks down and either too much fuel or not enough fuel is delivered to the cells that problems arise. All cells can "burn" glucose as a fuel. Most cells can utilize fat in an emergency. The glaring exception to this are the cells of the central nervous system, which include the brain. When the brain doesn't get enough glucose, it cannot function properly. When our brain cells cannot function properly, our behavior will be aberrant. It has to be, because our brains are running out of fuel!

In a healthy body, glucose is processed, refined, stored, and distributed to the waiting cells smoothly and efficiently. The amount in the bloodstream is regulated precisely and automatically. Those suffering from hypoglycemia, however, are not manifesting healthy bodies at this time and have temporarily lost their ability to perform this task. The mechanisms regulating the amount of blood sugar are defective, and the blood sugar is allowed to drop to dangerous levels.

But hypoglycemia is not an isolated symptom or group of symptoms. It is merely one way that our bodies can rebel when they have been denied nourishment (spiritual or physical). It indicates a body that is in need of help—not only a few isolated cells—but the whole body. The treatment, therefore, must be directed toward rehabilitating the whole body. We cannot mirror our perfect design for health until *all* our cells mirror that design.

The answer is to rehabilitate the body, especially the liver and pancreas, which are so vitally involved in blood sugar dynamics. This is done by changing the chemistry of the body—in other words, by eating properly and taking enough supplements for a long enough time to allow the body and these vital organs to regenerate themselves. This means that we will be establishing a whole new metabolism. It is almost like creating a whole new body. How exciting!

We rebuild the body into its perfect design with a complete nutritional program. We present to the cells every day all that they need in the form of the nutritional essentials. There is no taking of just one nutrient for one specific system. The body is one whole entity—a total system—and it must be treated as such.

Think Protein

In order to rebuild the body, the life force uses the amino acids present in all top-grade protein and restructures these amino acids into human tissue. Without proper protein, there is no maintenance, rebuilding, or renewing. So this is where our nutritional quest begins.

The ingestion of top-grade protein—the proper types in the proper amounts—cannot be overemphasized. In study after study it has been shown that the ingestion of many small high-protein meals throughout the day is one of the keys to controlling and overcoming low blood sugar.

The finest proteins are eggs, milk and milk products (such as yogurt, kefir, buttermilk, and others), cheese (including cottage cheese), fish, fowl, and lean meats. There are no finer single sources than these, and so they are the protein foods we should eat if we are looking for the finest health.

To assist the person manifesting hypoglycemia to determine if he has had sufficient protein, it may help to memorize this chart. The totals are approximate.

1 egg = 6 grams of protein
1 ounce of milk or milk product = 1 gram of protein
1 ounce of cheese = 7 grams (1 oz. cottage
     cheese = 4 grams)
1 ounce of fish, fowl, or lean meat = 5 grams

And what is a sufficient amount? Listen to your body to determine how much you need. We are all biochemically individual with individual needs. Generally speaking, however, you should try to ingest daily about one gram of protein for each two pounds of *ideal* body weight. (Please note that your *present* body weight may not be your *ideal* body weight!) If your ideal body weight is 120 pounds, for example, you will need about 60 grams of protein per day. You may find that while you are trying to overcome hypoglycemia you will need more. As has already been mentioned, the best way to do this is in many small meals. More about this later.

A special word about liver may be in order here. In a program designed to overcome a problem like hypoglycemia, the regular ingestion of liver can play a vital role. This is an amazing food—very high in protein, loaded with B vitamins (including high amounts of B12) and vitamin A, and containing energy-giving factors that have not yet been isolated. It can help strengthen our own livers. It helps overcome fatigue. It builds blood. Liver has provided many hypoglycemics with a new spark of energy and vitality. If possible, eat it several times a week. If you really don't like the taste, take desiccated liver tablets; but you will have to take many of them—10 or 15 or more a day—to accomplish noticeable good. (Desiccated liver is also available in powder form; but, if you don't like the taste of liver, you probably won't like the powder.) However you choose to take it, try to get some regularly. It can make a great difference in the way you feel.

Take Care with Carbohydrates

Carbohydrates are the fuel of the body. There is a danger inherent in all fuels, and carbohydrates are no exception. From carbohydrates we get most of the energy we need throughout the day. However, the ingestion of the wrong kinds of carbohydrates can present as explosive a situation in our bodies as can the burning of the wrong fuel in an engine.

We know that the secret of a good blood sugar level is in supplying the system with the proper nutrients, which will be broken down into glucose at the proper rate and in the proper amount. Sugar and anything containing sugar, white flour, and all refined carbohydrates and junk foods are *not* proper nutrients for the hypoglycemic or anyone else! It is also important to know that, when we eat foods that are too concentrated in sugar, the liver cannot process the sugar quickly enough. Excess sugar is dumped into the bloodstream and, much like kerosene reacts when dumped in a gently-burning coal fire, there is an explosion. Incineration figuratively rages in the body. Of course the body won't accept this situation, so the pancreas is alerted and secretes the hormone insulin, which results in lowering the blood sugar. The hardworking pancreas was not designed to combat such extremes, however; and, if this pattern is repeated too often over too many years, the pancreas reaches a state of exhaustion. In its attempt to reduce the blood sugar level it over-compensates and pulls the level down too far. This is when the hypoglycemic feels that awful slump with its attendant physical and emotional aberrations.

All carbohydrates stimulate insulin release. However, the more refined the carbohydrate the quicker the release. Sugar has the quickest and most dramatic effect. Our bodies were not designed to burn such high-powered fuels.

206

They were designed to utilize the complex or unrefined carbohydrates, breaking them down slowly so that the glucose is easily handled by the body.

The finest carbohydrates and the ones we should choose from are fresh fruits, fresh vegetables, and whole grains. That is it for the hypoglycemic! The list may seem short; but, when one considers all the wonderful fresh fruits, vegetables, and grains available, the list becomes full of many wonderful foods.

It might be best for hypoglycemics to keep away from fruit juices and dried fruit while they are rehabilitating the body. The natural sugar content in a glass of juice (which may contain the juice of 3 or 4 pieces of fruit or vegetable) may be much too high at this time. The same holds true with dried fruit which, because the moisture and therefore much of the volume has been removed, is much more concentrated in natural sugar than fresh fruit.

Those very sensitive hypoglycemics may not even be able to eat fresh fruit at this time. They will have to utilize more of the vegetables and grains until their "trigger happy" pancreas is further rehabilitated. You will have to experiment for yourself to see what works best.

Although oils do not have as specific an application as proteins and carbohydrates in the nutrition of the hypoglycemic, they are essential to good health because they are the only sources of essential fatty acids.

Some good oils are safflower oil, sunflower oil, corn oil, and more. Use these wonderful oils on salads and vegetables. Better Butter is great on toast.

Wheat germ oil is especially good. It is somewhat bitter and may not be a good choice to be used with foods. However, it can be put into a blender drink or taken in capsule form.

Other good sources of oil are raw nuts and seeds. Not only are they good sources of essential fatty acids but, because of their good protein content, they make great snacks. Eat them raw and unsalted or not at all.

In Addition to Food

Supplementing the diet with extra amounts of vitamins and minerals *after* embarking on a diet rich in top-grade proteins, constructive carbohydrates, and good oils is the next step toward the total renovation of the body temple. Remember, the body needs extra help or it would not be manifesting any malady. We should give it all the help it needs. If we present the body with abundant nutrients, it can choose what it needs and reject what it does not. If we don't present it with enough, it obviously cannot exercise this option.

A good way to initiate a supplementation of the diet is by taking a strong multiple vitamin-mineral containing all the vitamins (A, B complex, C, D, and E) and all the needed minerals. This is a minimum consideration and assures at least a minimum intake of all these nutrients. However, there is much reason to believe that one manifesting hypoglycemia may need much more than a minimum intake.

B Complex—In light of what was said about hypoglycemia being an indication of disturbed blood sugar dynamics, extra amounts of a strong B complex (all eleven B vitamins) would be in order. The B vitamins are very active in helping the body to metabolize carbohydrates by converting them into usable energy. Also, they are essential for the health of the nerves and can help us to better withstand stress. Both of these are areas in which the hypoglycemic needs help.

Vitamin C—This is really one of the "superstars" of nutrition. It is important for so many biochemical processes in the body. With regard to hypoglycemia, extra C is needed first of all because of its role in the health of the adrenal glands. Many hypoglycemics suffer from adrenal exhaustion; that is, their adrenal glands, which secrete the hormone adrenaline, are worn out from the continual stress which low blood sugar places on them.

Vitamin C is also important in fighting fatigue in the body, as it is essential for the absorption of iron and the utilization of important B vitamins that help prevent anemia.

The body cannot make its own vitamin C and must rely on outside sources to provide it. Many investigators suggest taking between 1,000 and 5,000 milligrams daily under normal conditions. Others think that the average is closer to 10,000 milligrams per day. Each of us, of course, must decide for himself.

Lipotropics—The liver is one of the key organs in maintaining health. This is especially true in overcoming hypoglycemia, for it is the liver that has much to do with processing, storing, and releasing glucose.

Although the cells of the liver have the potential to regenerate themselves indefinitely, when abused these cells begin filling up with fat and they die. Lipotropic agents are powerful fat movers and *in conjunction with* a total nutritional approach can rid the liver of this fat and regenerate the liver cells. It is not until the liver regains its health that we will regain ours.

Lipotropic formulas are usually a combination of one or more of the B complex vitamins *(choline, inositol,* and often *B12),* the amino acid *methionine* (present in all top-grade proteins) and often *betaine.*

Iron—Iron is an essential trace mineral because it is an integral part of the hemoglobin molecule and is most re-

sponsible for bringing oxygen to the cells. If your hypoglycemia has caused chronic fatigue, supplementation with a
good iron formula may be in order.

Breakfast—There are some special considerations that
the low blood sugar sufferer should take seriously. The first
is the importance of breakfast. Anyone suffering from hypoglycemia should never consider starting the day without the
proper breakfast. It would be like trying to begin a day's
drive without gasoline. We must eat well in the morning to
raise our blood sugar level for the day ahead. Good breakfast, good day. A good breakfast does not necessarily mean
a large breakfast; it means a breakfast with at least one top-
grade protein and one constructive carbohydrate. The addition of a good source of oil would make it even better. (In
addition to the typical breakfast fare of eggs and toast with
Better Butter, there are many other breakfasts that can be
eaten. How about some cottage cheese and fresh fruit for
breakfast? You might eat oatmeal or a granola-type cereal
with lots of milk. You might even eat a very lean ground
beef patty with some tomato. Use your imagination. Breakfast does not have to be boring or predictable.)

Small Meals—The ingestion of many small meals
throughout the day instead of three large ones does much
to help hypoglycemia since small meals do not "challenge"
the pancreas as do larger ones. Because of our life-styles it
is not always practical to eat this way, but whenever possible
it should be done. One way to do it is to eat a bit less at your
three meals and snack between meals on healthful things
like raw nuts and seeds or a piece of cheese and a quarter of
an apple, or a hard boiled egg and a slice of tomato, or a
glass of milk, or even a handful of desiccated liver tablets
with some tomato juice (with no sugar added!).

Brewer's Yeast—Chromium is a trace element in the
human body and is essential for carbohydrate metabolism.

In brewer's yeast, chromium appears at the center of a molecule known as the "glucose tolerance factor" (GTF). GTF works with insulin to maintain the delicate balance between *hypoglycemia* (*low* blood sugar) and *hyperglycemia* (*high* blood sugar). The fact that brewer's yeast is one of the best natural sources of GTF makes it a worthwhile special consideration for hypoglycemics. Brewer's yeast is available in tablet and powder form. It can bloat some people, so begin with small amounts. If you find that it continually bloats you, discontinue its use.

GTF chromium is available in tablet form for those who choose not to use brewer's yeast and for those who feel that they would like to have more of this special aid.

The Energizer—For those who would like to utilize small meals but whose life-styles are not compatible with this way of eating, a blender drink may be the solution. The authors have developed a high-protein, highly nutritious drink, which they call The Energizer. It can be made in the morning and put into a thermos to be sipped on throughout the day.

The Energizer (serves two meals)

Blend the following:

> 12 to 16 ounces of non-fat milk
> 1 or 2 raw eggs
> 1 teaspoonful wheat germ oil
> 1 heaping tablespoonful protein powder
> > (milk and egg type is best)
> 1 or 2 teaspoonful brewer's yeast
> 1 or 2 tablespoonful lecithin granules
> small piece of fresh fruit for taste.

This is a powerful drink so sip it S-L-O-O-O-W-L-Y; a few ounces at a time is a good amount. Take it with you to work and use it throughout the day to prevent a slump in energy.

(Brewer's yeast can cause excessive amounts of intestinal gas in some people. If you find this a problem after taking the drink for a few weeks, cut down on the amount of Brewer's yeast. If the problem persists, eliminate it entirely.)

Pancreatic Enzymes—Because there is truth to the adage that "like helps like," the use of digestive enzymes containing pancreatin can be of benefit to the pancreas. One or two tablets can be taken after each meal. These will also help you to properly digest the food.

Exercise—No regime of healthful rebuilding would be complete without regular exercise. It is natural to and needed by the body. In order for it to be effective, exercise should be done on a regular basis, preferably in the fresh air.

Exercise, in addition to being good for us physiologically, is good for us psychologically. It is most beneficial in calming the nerves. There is much evidence to show that the impulses generated in the spindles of the muscles during prolonged walking, for example, are essential to the proper functioning of our central nervous system.

Choose an exercise that suits you. Walking is always a good choice. Regular brisk walks are nature's antidote to stress. Also good are cycling, yoga, golf, horseback riding, and many others.

Avoid—There are certain things that the hypoglycemic should make every effort to avoid. In addition to the ones already mentioned, high on the list are smoking, drinking alcoholic beverages, the consumption of caffeine (coffee, tea, cola drinks, etc.) and other stimulants, high doses of estrogen, birth-control pills, excessive use of diuretics, and the foremost of these villains—stress.

Stress and anxiety can touch off severe low blood sugar. We know that in Truth nothing can harm us. All stress is actually self-induced. We are stressed not by situations themselves but by our *reactions* to situations. As we begin focusing our attention on our God—our good—our reactions will better mirror Him and stress will be a forgotten reaction, a thing of the past. But until that time, we must avoid situations that may lead to stress and keep rebuilding the body and soul, so that when these situations do arise, we are strong enough not to have them effect us.

Patience Brings Rewards

Cells that have been starved and mistreated may not seem to be responding immediately to your improved change of outlook, change of thoughts, and change of nutrition. Do not let this fact discourage you. When health has been coasting downhill for so long it may take awhile to reverse the trend and "gear-up" for the climb back toward health. But be sure of this: As soon as we begin seeking God, our health will improve. It will improve because *all* aspects of our lives will improve, including the thoughts we think and the foods we eat. Charles Fillmore once said: *Impurity is not altogether the result of the impure food that you eat. That has something to do with it, but the desire for impure food begins in the mind, a hungering of the impure thought for that whereon to feed and grow.*

When our thoughts are full of God and good, our actions will follow. When our actions are full of God and good, the renovation of our temples will be completed according to the exact blueprints of our perfection, and they will mirror their divine Architect as they were originally intended to do.

Handling High Blood Pressure

The veins and arteries are the mighty conduits through which the life-giving blood travels to every nook and cranny of the body temple. This bedazzling system of blood vessels is a network of almost unbelievable length—the capillaries alone, if stretched out end to end, would extend about 60,000 miles! That means there are about five yards of capillaries to each square inch of body surface! (No, that is not a misprint. It is just one more example of how truly *fearfully and wonderfully* we are made.)

The *contractibility* of these blood vessels is the key to normal blood pressure, a phenomenon that seems to be growing more and more rare these days. But this does not have to be the case at all. Could high blood pressure (hypertension) really be part of the divine plan for life? Could a Creator who seeks to express Himself through His human creations really condone brittle, inflexible arteries that are literally about as resilient as a dried-out inner tube? It doesn't make sense, does it? Then why is there such a pervasive incidence of this degenerative condition? Let's see if we can discover the answer to these questions.

In order to make our bodies as foolproof as possible, God designed them in a most ingenious way. Ninety-nine percent of the bodily functions are outside our conscious control. And it's a good thing they are! God knew what He was doing when He put the functions of all the major glands and organs in the all-knowing hands of the life force as it operates independently of our conscious thought. Can you imagine what a state of chaos we would be in if we had to consciously control the beating of the heart, the pumping of the blood, the work of the lungs, the digestion and assimilation of foods, the converting of nutrients into new tissue, the secretion of hormones and enzymes, the excretion of wastes—oh, the list is staggering! We all know that such a responsibility would be unthinkable—impossible.

But not to the divine life force! It knows exactly what to do and how to do it—if we let it! God did give us one marvelous gift. This gift enables us to reach the pinnacles of Christhood or sink to such depths of physical wreckage that, as Charles Fillmore puts it: . . . *in the end [we] dump the old "boat" at the junk pile.*

What is this most awesome of gifts? Our willpower— our free will—our ability to decide for ourselves the outcome of our lives. Free will invests us with the power to set causes into motion. It means, by the same token, that we must take full responsibility for the effects those causes inevitably bring to us.

What has this to do with high blood pressure? Everything! It means that we have exercised our freedom of will in ways that might not have been the most prudent in the long run. It means that over the years we might not always have made the right choices regarding our spiritual, mental, and physical nourishment. But it also means that we are free to turn this will right around and put into motion an entirely new set of causes—causes that will bring us a new spectrum of effects more to our liking. Normal blood pressure will be just such an effect. The point is that the choice is ours. If we don't like something about our lives, we have the power to change it.

Before we can change anything, however, we have to know what it is we are changing and how to go about doing it, don't we? Since we have a three-fold nature—Spirit, soul, and body—we will naturally examine each of these

215

aspects to discover some causes as well as some "cures."

Spirit first. Always Spirit first. This is the essence of our lives, the Christ-perfect pattern built into each of us. Our destiny must be to align ourselves completely with this indwelling Christ ideal so that our bodies and minds will become one with the idea of total perfection.

The way to oneness is the way of meditation and prayer. To many of us it seems that Spirit is an abstract concept—untouchable and unknowable. But this is not true. We discover that as we wind our way inward we are filled with the joy of the approaching encounter with the only thing that is truly real—the activity of Spirit, of the life force, as it shines forth from the center of our beings. It becomes knowable and touchable as we attune ourselves to it. We must be aware of the activity of God within us. It is the only power at work, and when we put our faith in it and flow with it we can expect to experience untold changes in our lives.

There is work to be done in the mental realm. The consciousness must be conditioned to repel negativity and admit into its inner sanctum only positive, health-producing thoughts and beliefs. This requires practice, but it must be done if we are to achieve the right soil from which to grow healthy bodies.

We need to root out old attitudes of unforgiveness. We need to soften our hardened, brittle attitudes if we want to soften our hardened, brittle arteries! We must probe our minds and hearts for any such encumbrances and release them at once. We have no need of them.

The relaxation attained during meditation is a perfect opportunity to rid ourselves of stress, which is a major contributor to hypertension. We physically and mentally relax, loosing and letting go of all burdens, as we speak words of health to our priceless blood vessels. See them as pliant, resilient, and strong as they ceaselessly go about their task of directing the red sea of life through the body temple. We can encourage them and praise them and know that they are perfect.

Physical Foes

If we continually seek spiritual oneness with the life force and daily set aside time for meditation, it will be natural for us to want to learn and obey God's laws for the body temple.

It has been said that strong, resilient arteries are the most accurate physical signs of youthfulness. If this is true, it behooves us to know not only the rules involved in caring for these arteries but the list of various assailants to them as well. *High blood pressure . . . is most frequently a sign of auto-intoxication (a result of poor elimination), tension, protracted worry, fatigue, tobacco, alcohol stimulants, and lack of mineral-rich, vitamin-rich foods. Generally several of these factors are to blame.* This quote is from John Loughran's book "The Bionomy of Power." Similar indictments of those factors that contribute to hypertension can be found in almost any standard medical textbook.

Other culprits are sodium chloride (table salt) and spices. It is best to avoid both as much as possible. Human basic requirements for sodium are around 200 milligrams per day—that's the amount of sodium in about one-tenth teaspoonful of salt. Under the most extreme circumstances, not more than 2,000 mgs. is needed—about 1 teaspoonful. Yet Americans, on the average, ingest between 6,000 and 15,000 mgs. of sodium per day, not including snacks! This will not surprise you when you realize that sodium is present in our diets in more than ordinary table salt—sodium chloride. Other sodium sources in food are sodium-containing additives such as baking soda (sodium bicarbonate), monosodium glutamate (MSG), brine (table salt and water), disodium phosphate, sodium proprionate, and sodium sulfite.

Of course, when we eat a good balance of natural, un-processed, unrefined foods, we almost automatically eat the proper ratio of sodium and potassium. When food is processed, the sodium is almost always too high and the potassium too low. For example, whereas one spear of fresh asparagus contains 1 mg. of sodium, one spear of the canned variety has 74 mgs.; a cup of fresh lima beans con-tains 2 mgs. of sodium, the same amount of canned has 456 mgs. A typical serving of canned soup may contain more than 1,000 mgs. of sodium!

While the sodium and potassium are in a special bal-ance in a healthy body, in one suffering from high blood pressure this balance may be disturbed with sodium far in excess of the proper ratio. In such a case, it is imperative to realign that balance. The absolute amount of each is not as important as the crucial ratio between them. The intake of sodium should be restricted and potassium should be in-creased. If you are having trouble restricting your salt in-take, the best way to begin is to use a mixture of potassium chloride (K salt) and sodium chloride for seasoning, and to eat a good amount of fresh fruits and vegetables high in potassium. Some good ones are melons, bananas, winter squash, strawberries, oranges, peaches, dried fruit, and many more.

Actually we obtain ample natural sodium from our foods without having to add salt to them. Many people find that their taste buds will change and that they gradually learn to enjoy the natural *true* flavor of foods that have not been salted. This usually takes a month or so. (If you decide to cut down on your salt intake with the intention of finally eliminating it, you should be aware that the popular sea salt is still sodium chloride and would not belong in your diet. There are a few excellent vegetable "salts" available that are not very high in sodium. Read the labels carefully.)

The importance of this sodium-potassium balance or ratio is demonstrated by Dr. Hugh C. Trowell, a physician and teacher in Kenya for thirty years. There he saw people move from tribal diets to rapid westernization in eating habits. During this time the incidence of high blood pressure went from almost nil to become a common malady of Kenyans. The long experience that Dr. Trowell had with observing the change in the health of the Kenyans as their diets became more westernized led him to state: *. . . by reversing the high sodium to low potassium ratio of our Western diet, and of dietary fiber, over half of the people suffering from essential hypertension will achieve normal blood pressure in a few weeks.*

Spices that are hot to the taste raise the blood pressure. (They are also irritants to the delicate body tissues, which is a reason that *everyone* should avoid them.)

Junk foods and refined carbohydrates are detrimental to the blood pressure. Here is another quote from "The Bionomy of Power": *The essence of diet planning in high blood pressure is to enrich the diet with minerals and vitamins and to sharply decrease the refined foods (such as white flour and . . . sugar items) that tend to make a carbohydrate "glue" the ultimate effect of which is to "petrify" the tissue and hasten the process of hardening the arteries. It is important in blood vascular tension that tea and coffee be reduced to a minimum. Tobacco must be ruled out at once without any nonsense about "tapering off." All forms of smoking are herewith included and their discontinuance must be at once and complete, and, it may be added, permanent.*

219

Physical Friends

You have heard about the arterial foes. Hear now about the arterial friends—the benefactors of the divine life force. We should become thoroughly familiar with them.

The life force within us looks to the food we eat in order to obtain the building materials with which to fashion our bodies. It can use no other raw materials. It is important therefore that our diets be as rich as possible in essential nutrients so that the tissues fashioned will be of the finest quality.

Good nutrition begins with good food, and good food begins with good protein. We will not succeed physically without good protein, for maintaining, rebuilding, and re-newing tissue are impossible without it.

The finest protein foods are eggs, milk and milk products, cheese (including cottage cheese), fish, fowl, and lean meats. There are no finer single sources of protein than these. (Please see chapter two, page 17, for more information concerning protein.)

The next consideration in a healthful diet should be that of choosing a good constructive carbohydrate. (See chapter two, pages 20-22, for further information.)

Oils are the third nutritional essential as far as food is concerned. Our bodies have a need for essential fatty acid, and oils are the only foods where these are available. Choose a pleasant-tasting oil like safflower oil, sunflower oil, corn oil, or any of the other good ones. (Pages 22-25)

Other sources of good oil are nuts and seeds. These are best eaten raw and *unsalted*.

One helpful hint about eating: Try to eat many small meals instead of a few large ones. The ingestion of large meals can put a greater strain on the heart and blood vessels.

There is much evidence to conclude that, when we are trying to overcome a specific problem in the body, foods alone may not supply us with enough nutrients to overcome that problem completely. We may need many times the amount of certain nutrients than we normally would.

Such being the case, it would be wise to include in our daily intake a multiple vitamin-mineral formula of high potency. This formula should contain strong amounts of vitamins A, D, E, B complex, and C, as well as the essential minerals. Although we may need more of certain of these, this formula taken daily will assure at least a minimum intake of most of them.

Statistics show that as we get older we tend to show a greater deficiency in minerals. We know that age itself cannot be responsible for anything, but if we have eaten poorly for most of our lives, then age has given us more time to nutritionally abuse ourselves. Since minerals can be in short supply in the foods we normally eat, even if chosen carefully, it may be wise to add a separate multiple mineral tablet.

Again, this is a form of nutritional insurance. If we present the body with an abundance of nutrients, it will pick and choose what it needs and reject what it does not need. If we present it with too few nutrients, it obviously does not have this option.

The B complex vitamins are involved in so many aspects of food metabolism, energy production, and hundreds of other processes in the body that even a small deficiency can cause problems. Sufficient B complex vitamins are also needed for the health of the heart and blood vessels. You will probably want to add a strong B complex (all eleven of the B vitamins) to your daily dietary regime.

Vitamin C and a closely related substance which is part of the vitamin C "complex," bioflavonoids, are essential for the health of the blood vessels. They act together to add strength and resiliency to the blood vessel walls. Therefore, it would be a good idea to consider taking extra amounts of these two important vitamins. They can be purchased together in one tablet and are also available separately.

There are some special aids that have proven useful by many in the treatment of high blood pressure. Keep in mind that all of these special aids are subordinate to the good, solid laws of total nutrition. And the laws of nutrition are subordinate to thoughts of God and good.

Lecithin—Because we are dealing with a problem that often involves the obstruction of the blood vessels with unnatural fatty deposits, it would be helpful if we could remove those deposits and allow the blood to flow more freely and therefore at a lower pressure. Because of its soap-like characteristics, lecithin is a powerful emulsifying agent, and its presence in the blood tends to dissolve cholesterol deposits. It has proved in many studies to play a major role in maintaining the clarity of the blood system.

Lecithin is available in liquid, capsule, and granular form—the latter being the most potent and economical. The ingestion of a tablespoonful or more a day of this fine, harmless substance might go a long way toward rehabilitating and maintaining our health.

Lipotropics—Lecithin can also be made in our bodies. We can help to promote its synthesis by assuring the presence in our diets of the B complex vitamins choline and inositol, and the amino acid methionine (found in all top-grade protein). These are three lipotropic agents, and they are also useful in the detoxification of our hard-working liver. Lipotropics can be purchased in combined form in a single tablet.

There are several other suggestions to be made for hypertension. You might want to try some or all of them.

Garlic has traditionally been used to help lower elevated blood pressure and has proved to be effective in some cases. Capsules of garlic oil are probably the most convenient (and least offensive to others!) means of taking it.

As a beverage, raspberry leaf tea can be tried. This is the herbal tea most similar in taste to "real" tea, incidentally.

Such cultured foods as yogurt and acidophilus are influential in establishing the correct bacteria population in the large intestine. These friendly bacteria help keep down the count of the harmful bacteria, which is one of the causes of certain types of high blood pressure.

Raw unprocessed bran is another aid to the intestines if there is a problem with elimination. Remember that poor elimination can lead to auto-intoxication, which we already know to be a contributor to high blood pressure.

And then there is yucca, a desert plant that has been proven beneficial by at least one team of researchers. Reporting their results in the "Journal of Applied Nutrition," Doctors Bingham, Harris, and Laga had this to say: *Yucca extract, in tablet or liquid form, is recommended as a safe and effective food supplement to reduce abnormal levels of blood triglycerides and blood cholesterol and to lower abnormal blood pressure.* They hastened to add, however, that: *. . . all patients were placed on high-protein diets with natural foods, and they were given exercise programs and vitamin supplements.*

Which brings us to the final friend in our quest for perfection—exercise. No regime of total health is complete without regular exercise. One that can be done in the fresh air and sunshine would be best. Regular brisk walks are of course ideal, but also good are cycling, swimming, yoga, and many, many others. Choose the right one for you and do it regularly. Any program designed to rebuild human tissue must incorporate regular exercise.

True to Ourselves

The doctors who performed the experiment with yucca tablets made an important point when they reminded us that their patients were first put on a proper regime of total nutrition and good exercise.

We in the Truth movement would take it one crucial step further. To have a complete and permanent healing there have to be not only *total* nutrition and adequate regular exercise, but there must be a change of consciousness as well. It is in the spiritual realm that genuine healing takes place. If we are true to ourselves by being true to the great life force within us, we will be living lives of dedication to all three aspects of our being—Spirit, soul, and body. That is how healing comes about: That is how hypertension is overcome.

Pregnancy—Passport for a Soul

What in all of human experience could be more creative or wonder-filled than bringing a new life into the world? Imagine, a soul is embodying through you! You have been chosen to be the means of entrance into creation of a new being. Truly it is a time to sing as did Mary the mother of Jesus: . . . *"My soul magnifies the Lord, and my spirit rejoices in God my Savior."* (Luke 1:46, 47)

What a most special time, this time of pregnancy. Beginning with a single cell the life force goes mysteriously about its work of fashioning, according to a divine blueprint, a living human being. As the tiny cells multiply they silently differentiate into specialized tissue—some to form the nervous system, some to form the miniature heart, some to bud into diminutive fingers, and some to become baby seashell ears.

It all takes place in a grand and heavenly order, and the miracle of it all is that it is entirely directed by the universal life force which knows precisely what to do. This life force not only has the idea and desire to create a new life, it also has the means of doing it.

During the nine months in the womb, babies are in a state of continual change and growth and are more affected by the environment than they ever will be again in their entire lives. What happens in that watery cradle determines much concerning the eventual states of soul and physical health. That is why prospective mothers should devote themselves to providing the best environments for their unborn children.

Truly it is a blessed privilege to prepare for the coming into the physical of a soul . . . , wrote Myrtle Fillmore. *Just now, especially, you do not want to worry or be anxious for the future. You want your mind and your body calm and peaceful and happy, so that you will be radiating only the best and most helpful things to your unborn babe. Your own attitude is imparting qualities to the soul of your child.*

So just make up your mind that you are going to live in a little world all your own, a world of beauty, and peace, and happiness, and health, and simple pleasures. (These words are from *Myrtle Fillmore's Healing Letters.* Any prospective parent would derive much inspiration and direction from the chapter entitled "Maternity.")

The nine months preceding birth provide the opportunity for helping a soul to achieve its best development. It asks to be allowed to be its true self. It desires happiness, peace, and health. It longs for the companionship of wise and loving parents. The life inside the womb may be a dark and solitary one, but it is nonetheless a feeling one—a perceptive and receptive one. It is being "programmed" for its future all that time—a future that you, as the bearer of that soul, have the power to help shape.

Your responsibility to your unborn child lies in two major areas: spiritual and physical. Let us consider the spiritual first, since it is the basis for all else.

Nurture the Arriving Soul

As you do not know how the spirit comes to the bones in the womb of a woman with child, so you do not know the work of God who makes everything. (Eccles. 11:5) It is true that, while we cannot fathom the deep mysteries of the workings of Spirit—how it builds a human being out of a single cell—we do see the evidence of those workings. We feel the presence of Spirit and are awed by its creative power.

The expectant mother can put her baby into the care and protection of the Almighty. She can speak words of peace and love to the life growing within her, trusting in the goodness of God and affirming to that little life words about " . . . *the Lord who made you, who formed you from the womb and will help you.*" (Isa. 44:2)

Nothing should be permitted to disturb the atmosphere of joy and serenity and harmony which provides the ideal spiritual environment for the emerging soul. What better way for that soul to establish a firm footing in spiritual strength than to spend nine months in such an environment?

At this time also the prospective parents should be envisioning a perfect baby, sound in every way. Words can be spoken directly to the life force as it goes about its work within the womb. What a beautiful and creative experience it is to participate in the building of a new life. And this is the priceless opportunity each prospective parent has. Make each of those 270 days count, nurturing that soul with your finest spiritual gifts. It is probably not humanly possible to know the extent to which you can permanently affect the thinking and feeling nature of that burgeoning soul with your own thoughts and feelings during the gestation period. This aspect should be always foremost in your mind.

Nurture the Tiny Body

The second major area of responsibility to the unborn child is that of physical welfare—physical health. The role of nutrition is crucial. As nutrition counselors, the authors are frequently asked at what point should good nutrition be put into practice in order to provide optimum nourishment for

227

the developing fetus. The answer—and not one to be taken lightly—is: two years before conception, on the part of both parents!

Nature, in its inimitable way, will always strive to provide the best nutrients and building materials for the fetus. The state of health of both parents at the time of conception, along with the continuing state of health of the pregnant mother, determines greatly the quality of health being built into that baby. If there is a low quality to the nutrition of the parents before conception and a low quality to that of the mother during pregnancy, there is little with which the life force can work.

Abundant nutrients have to be available to the fetus for growth to proceed normally. As ingenious as the life force is, it cannot do much to build strength and integrity into the unborn tissues if there is a paucity of nutrients with which to work. It is of strategic importance, therefore, that much effort be devoted to proper nutrition during (and before!) pregnancy. Your child's physical future depends upon it.

The proper diet will include wholesome foods, vitamins, and minerals. There will be no junk foods because you do not want a baby with "junk food tissues," do you? The proper diet creates a favorable environment for prenatal growth. An improper diet does not. Things like tobacco, alcohol, stimulant drugs, diuretic drugs, tranquilizers, dieting (with or without the use of amphetamine-containing appetite suppressors) have no place in the designing of a new life, and would only serve to seriously endanger that life's chances for perfection.

"A Physician's Handbook on Orthomolecular Medicine" emphasizes how important good nutrition is: *In a world where suboptimal nutrition generally prevails, pregnant women are often inadequately nourished. Nature tries to provide growing fetuses with good environments, but it is powerless to do so if the necessary raw materials are absent from the food consumed.* Are the necessary raw materials absent from *your* diet? Just what are these necessary raw materials?

The Nutritional Environment

The prime concern is protein, because it is required in the building of all of the new little tissues. Protein is the stuff of which our bodies and babies' bodies are made, and the prospective mother should be sure to eat enough of it. Eggs, milk and milk products, cheese (including cottage cheese), lean meat, fish, and poultry are the best sources of protein. It would be advisable to eat at least one selection from that list at every meal, including snacks. (If you prefer not to eat any animal products at all, it is possible to obtain a good grade of protein by skillfully combining your other foods. However, you must be knowledgeable in your combinations so that you get the best amino acid content and balance.)

You will need to eat *good* carbohydrates. (The world abounds in bad ones!) This means fresh fruits, fresh vegetables, whole grains (including a good whole-grain bread), and, if you need to sweeten something, honey, blackstrap molasses, or pure maple syrup. For your own sake and that of your baby, no sugar or white flour, nor any of the multitude of fake foods into which these "bad news" items are incorporated should be eaten. Even a little bit hurts. It is not worth it.

Third on the list of foods is oil. You may need a teaspoonful or more of a good, cold-pressed vegetable oil each day. Safflower, corn, sunflower, or sesame are good choices. If you will take wheat germ oil or cod liver oil, so much the better. The body temple—born and unborn—re-

229

quires essential fatty acids. We obtain these from our good oils and from the nuts and seeds containing these oils.

Good vitamin supplementation is important during pregnancy. Make sure that you have the complete B complex (eleven B vitamins) in your formula. All the vitamins are needed, of course. Good amounts of vitamin C may also be helpful.

In addition to the B complex, many studies have shown that additional amounts of B6 can be of great benefit, especially in relieving the nausea which often accompanies pregnancy.

Most prospective mothers are aware of their great need for calcium. It is required for building the bones and teeth of the baby; it can prevent leg cramps in the mother; and it is necessary for numerous functions in the body of both mother and child. A good calcium supplement is a good investment in the health of two people, since it is very difficult to obtain the appropriate amounts of this major mineral from foods alone. Calcium can be taken after each meal and again at bedtime.

But don't forget, the body needs all the other major and trace minerals if it is to express its perfection and if it is to help the fetus fulfill its grand design. Let's be sure that the diet is rich in mineral-containing foods—unrefined foods. If it is not, then a mineral supplement may be in order.

Exercise Required

In any program designed to create good health, exercise is a necessary adjunct. Your physician will no doubt suggest the types of physical exercise best suited to your needs. Perhaps taking your baby for a walk every day before it is born would be good.

Whatever exercise you decide is best for you and the

unborn baby should be done regularly. Motion is part of the law. We must move in order to improve.

Learn the spiritual and physical laws required for building a body temple. These laws were ordained by the Master Temple Builder. When we awaken to the wonders of life and the miracle of birth, we become filled with the desire to serve the life force which directs it all. We come to love the law because we see that by adhering to it we open the pathway to perfection, both spiritual and physical. We come to see that the law of God makes provisions for all things, even the intricate sculpturing of a tiny new life. Our delight, like the Psalmist's, should be in the law of the Lord. *O, how I love thy law! It is my meditation all the day.* (Psalms 119:97)

Loving the Law

True concern for the law—allowing it to operate in the spiritual and physical development of the unborn babe—will bring a new sense of joy and peace into your own life. And it will provide an atmosphere of splendor for the growing fetus, guiding it perfectly to the day when that soul makes its triumphant entry into this beautiful, Christ-lit world.

That soul selected *you*. It needs your help and your love. Its spiritual and physical nourishment are in your hands. What an opportunity! What a privilege! What a blessing!

Strong Bones for Sturdy Temples

Uncounted ages before the architects of Rome swung the first dome atop the Pantheon and built arches to support the aqueducts, the dome of the skull already roofed the human head in its present perfection, the arches of the foot provided a strong, springy support for the body's weight in motion, and the arched ribs formed a light, flexible cage sheltering the organs of the thorax. The columns of the Greeks and Egyptians were antedated by the columns of animals and human legs, and the first curved portal in man's experience was the gateway of the pelvis through which he entered the world.

Those beautiful lines from "Man and His Body" by Benjamin Miller, MD, and Ruth Goode give us a sense of appreciation for the wonder of our skeletal system—our bones. The bones of the human body are an encyclopedia of mechanical and architectural principles which serve as the basis for much of our modern engineering science. The strength of concrete blocks and hollow bricks is patterned after the Haversian canals of our long bones (the birthplace of our blood cells), and the spans of bridges, levers, and cantilevers are patterned after our phenomenal joints.

All architectural plans that make the skyscraper possible, all the dreams and love that go into the making of a house are comparatively nothing when you think of the divine wisdom that planned the framework of your body, the love that called it forth, the workmanship that became manifest in it, and the ever-renewing life that was built into every supporting or protective bone.

The very life and substance of God permeate your bones. His strength supports them. They give stability to the whole structure of your body, protect and shelter its vital organs, and preserve its shape, says Clara Palmer in *You Can Be Healed.*

Think of the work that went into your bones—their design and their strength. And think what you would look like without them! You would resemble nothing more than a shapeless mass of jelly. We *need* our bones to give us our distinctly human form.

There was no hit-or-miss work to this design. Each bone has the exact strength, size, and location for its use. It was planned within your tissues before you were born. These cells knew to convert their soft tissues into hard bones long before they would be put to actual use. The great Mind within them silently carried out its prophetic structuring, ever-toiling toward the ultimate goal: that of a complete and perfect human being.

Time Is Not Our Enemy

When one considers the mighty creative work undertaken by the life force on behalf of our noble skeletal system, it would seem like heresy, would it not, to ever regard weak, distorted, or crumbling bones as normal?

Too often we fall victim to the old race belief that the older one gets the more fragile become his bones. We are told we just have to accept the "fact" and live with it. Ridiculous! Would this be the plan of an almighty Creator whose works are only for the good? Let us see what the real facts are.

One of the essential constituents of bones is the mineral calcium. Our body uses calcium every second and we lose some every day. Regardless of age, the body loses calcium. According to Dr. Leo Litwak, professor of medicine at the School of Medicine, University of California at Los Angeles, about 1,000 milligrams of calcium are needed daily to prevent osteoporosis (soft bones) and effectively replace the calcium lost each day in the urine, digestive juices, perspiration, feces, and muscle movement. We need calcium for so very many functions of the body that it must be continually replaced. The body does not make its own minerals; it must rely on an outside source for them. That is why we must make sure of a good supply of calcium every day.

Right Use of Time

Can you see the picture? It is not age that weakens bones through loss of calcium. It is not because we are sixty or eighty or ninety years old. How could years possibly hurt us? They are only a limited form of measurement. They tell us how many times we have traveled around the sun. Therefore, years and ages are unimportant in themselves.

What *is* important is the use we have made of that time. Have we invested it wisely in good eating habits, plenty of exercise, and right spiritual progress? Have we used that time as an opportunity to replace the vital nutrients that are necessary for the proper functioning of the miraculous body? If we have, if we have adhered to the inviolable laws God provided so that we can maintain our temples as He desires us to, we can expect healthy, strong bones—the kind referred to in Job 40:18: *"His bones are tubes of bronze. . . . "* Why settle for less? We don't have to, and certainly we're not supposed to.

The only unchanging aspect of the human body is change itself. Bones are no exception. Radioactive isotopes introduced into the body for the purpose of experimentation have been detected going into and out of the bones. In other words, bones exchange their structure hour by hour. Whereas it was once thought that bone minerals could not be replaced, we now know that we are constantly building new skeletons. This means that we can take advantage of this fact and see to it that we build good ones. Then: *. . . your heart shall rejoice; your bones shall flourish like the grass. . . .* (Isaiah 66:14)

Calcium for Strength

We have already said that in order to have good bones, whether we are maintaining them or regenerating them, we need a good intake of calcium. Milk and milk products, including cheese, yogurt, etc., are good food sources of this most important mineral, as are shellfish, egg yolks, canned sardines (with bones), and many green leafy vegetables. But, unless we are absolutely certain that we are obtaining ample amounts from them, it seems advisable to supplement the diet with some good calcium tablets. Perhaps you might take some bone meal—a good source of calcium, as well as phosphorus, which is also essential for the bones and teeth.

Let us remember that the body, like everything else, is designed and functions on the principle of unity. Everything is interrelated. Therefore, calcium alone, while extremely important, will not build strong bones and teeth.

Protein a Primary Consideration

Protein is the major organic material with which God has chosen to construct our skeletal systems. We should try to obtain some form of complete top-grade protein at each meal. These top-grade proteins include eggs, milk, cheese, fish, fowl, and lean meat. Please note that you do not have to eat all these foods. Some may not want to eat meat, others may not like milk or eggs or cheese. However, it is usually best if you choose your protein from this list. These foods are known as "complete" proteins and contain an optimum balance of the essential amino acids—the building blocks needed to build and repair human tissue. In other words, these foods, even when eaten alone, will supply the raw materials needed for bodily repair and renewal.

Grains, nuts, seeds, vegetables, and fruits also contain protein, and it is possible to be perfectly healthy eating them and not eating the top-grade proteins previously mentioned. However, a word of warning is in order. These individual non-animal proteins are usually incomplete or unbalanced in their amino acid content. Therefore, when they are eaten alone they cannot be relied on to supply the proper balance of amino acids. It is important, therefore, to learn how to combine them to optimize the amino acid pattern.

Only protein contains the amino acids which, by ingenious design, are reassembled into human tissue. Most of us do not eat enough protein to rebuild and renew ourselves. Obtaining sufficient amounts of top-grade protein in our daily diets is the first nutritional essential in rebuilding healthy bones.

We also need a good carbohydrate at each meal. Select one or more fresh fruits, vegetables, or whole grains (which may be in the form of a whole-grain bread, granola, etc.). And, if a sweetener is needed, use only small amounts of honey, blackstrap molasses, or pure maple syrup. (Sugar, white flour, and all junk foods have no place in the body temple.)

The important thing is to ingest a *good* carbohydrate. If we don't eat some carbohydrate, which will be used as fuel, the body will resort to burning its protein in order to obtain the needed fuel. And we do not want to sacrifice our vital building materials that way.

Cod Liver Oil

The third food type we need is oil. Like all machines, the miracle machine that we are needs a good oil. The wonderful vegetable oils like safflower oil, corn oil, sesame oil, and others are marvelous choices, and because of their taste are fine for use with salads, on baked potatoes, on toast, and in cooking. But, in dealing with health of the bones, there is one oil that has a very special significance. That oil is cod liver oil, a marvelous aid to the bones because it is very rich in vitamin D. Without this important vitamin we are unable to absorb the calcium that we ingest.

Although a healthy body can make vitamin D from sunlight, a teaspoonful of cod liver oil each day will do much to ensure healthy bones. Luckily cod liver oil can be obtained in flavored form, and it is also available in capsule form. No matter how you obtain it, be sure that it is part of your nutritional regime.

Of course, the body temple requires all the many nutrients in existence. That is why a good multiple vitamin supplement, containing the complete (all eleven) B complex, is a minimum precaution worth taking. Why deprive the life force of what it needs for maximum performance? And who knows what maximum is! Our spiritual and physical potentials are both still relatively unexplored.

Vitamin C deserves some special mention here because it is so necessary for strong bones. It is also necessary for strong connective tissue, blood vessels, gums, and, believe it or not, spinal disks. These disks are actually collagenous cushions between the vertebrae and respond beautifully to large amounts of vitamin C, along with adequate amounts of the other important nutrients.

Lack of vitamin C causes bones to show a lattice-like or ground-glass appearance under X-ray. Vitamin C, then, is a key factor in building strong bones. Scientists doing the research on this versatile nutrient indicate that, because we cannot make it in our bodies, our needs are greater than formerly thought, with most of us not getting anywhere near what we should from our food.

A Helpful Hint

Try supplementing your diet with optimum amounts of vitamin C. And what is your optimum amount? That is something only you can decide. The Recommended Daily Allowance (RDA) of the Food and Nutrition Board tells us that about seventy-five milligrams of vitamin C should be sufficient each day. Many other scientists find this suggestion much too low. Men of the caliber of Dr. Linus Pauling (Noble Prize-winning chemist) and Dr. Albert Szent-Györgyi (the discoverer of vitamin C and also a Nobel Prize-winning chemist) reason that the optimum amount of this crucial vitamin is closer to between 1,000 and 5,000 milligrams per day—and could even be as high as 10,000 milligrams per day.

If you are not getting results with the amount of vitamin C you are now taking, you could try taking more.

We have been discussing some of the beneficial nutrients in the building of healthy bones. Let's take a minute to mention something *not* so beneficial. Many people take antacid products for their stomachs, when they should be taking a good digestive enzyme or some hydrochloric acid (HCl) tablets. Hydrochloric acid occurs naturally in our stomachs and is needed to prepare calcium for proper absorption. Antacid preparations are not the answer to many digestive problems, nor are they necessarily advisable for people who want healthier bones.

The stomach antacid, aluminum hydroxide gel, which has many trade names, can greatly reduce blood phosphate. . . . With low serum (blood) phosphate the bones dissolve, the muscles ache and are extremely weak. . . . Older patients, who are particularly subject to osteoporosis (loss of calcium in the bones), should therefore limit the use of aluminum hydroxide gel.

This advice is from the renowned head of the Brain-Bio Center at Princeton, New Jersey, Carl C. Pfeiffer, PhD, MD, in his book "Mental and Elemental Nutrients." Perhaps what he said may be of interest to you. Only you can determine this for sure.

The works and workings of God are for the most part beyond our comprehension. We do not understand *how* it all works, but we have come to discover the principles by which it does work.

Exercise — Part of the Law

We don't really know the secrets by which the mighty cell converts food to living flesh, but we do know what nutrients are required to do the job. We also know that physical exercise is required of us. There are some important reasons that exercise is crucial to good bone health.

One reason is our constant need for calcium. We cannot afford to lose any. Our bones and muscles (and don't forget that the heart is a muscle) must have calcium in order to function according to their divine plan. Exercise helps us maintain calcium. After only three days of inactivity, the bones begin to lose their supply. That is why long durations of bed rest are generally not good and begin to weaken the

239

body temple. Calcium is lost from the bones. The astronauts on an eight-day mission in space lost 200 milligrams of calcium daily, in spite of their exercise program. Because of their weightlessness, they simply could not get the type of physical activity necessary to maintain proper calcium levels.

Exercise, then, must be a part of our temple renovation project. We live in a universe of motion. We are designed to move, and move we must if we are to improve the quality and quantity of our lives.

Choose an exercise appropriate for you. Walking, jogging, swimming, yoga, and bicycling are but a few of the host of wonderful exercises you can do to strengthen your muscles and bones.

Integrate one or more of these exercises into your lifestyle. How about walking to the store next time instead of taking the car? Or, when you go shopping, why not use the stairs instead of the elevator? How about using your bicycle to go to the newspaper stand each day instead of riding in an automobile? Remember, regular movement will lead to improvement.

Malstructure Means Malfunction

There is another vital reason for exercising. It pertains to the structure of the temple itself. (We must remember that form and function are indivisible.) Let us regress for a moment and remind you that red blood cells are formed in the marrow of the bones. Keep this fact in mind, now, as we look at posture and exercise.

If there are structural inbalances in the anatomy, blood vessels are impinged on and free blood flow inhibited. Malstructure then leads to malfunction. In this respect, posture is crucial. The alignment of neck, shoulders, and backbone should be carefully checked.

It is not unusual that, as we gain years, we lose height. The back of the neck curves inward too far, throwing the head forward. The upper back becomes too rounded and humped, crowding the ribs. The lower back grows swayed. This describes people all about us, doesn't it?

These tendencies can and must be counteracted with correct posture and exercises because there is more than the skeletal structure involved. Physiologists discovered that we initially produce red blood cells in the marrow of all bones. As we slow down our physical activity, the long bones (such as the femur or thigh bone) stop making these red cells. It becomes obvious that these long bones need the stimulation of vigorous use.

Bones do respond to muscular activity, and when they do not get it, the marrow loses its ability to manufacture healthy red blood cells. Production is then turned over to the vertebrae, ribs, breastbone, and other flat bones. These bones must be stimulated by exercise or they are unable to carry on with their work. Red cell production will decrease, and anemia can result.

Can you see the importance of correct posture and exercise? The body temple must be straight and properly aligned. Who would want to build a church with sagging, crooked walls?

Meaning of Bones

There are metaphysical aspects of the bones that we must examine. Clara Palmer in *You Can Be Healed* writes: *Your bones, the framework and support of your body, symbolize your substance and stability in Truth.* Are we thoroughly grounded—firmly rooted—in Truth? The foundation must be solid, for upon it we build all else.

241

Because God is mentioned at the end of this chapter is not to demean the importance of the spiritual. In fact, quite the opposite is true. As in every aspect of our lives, we must put God first. . . . *fear the Lord, and turn away from evil. It will be . . . refreshment to your bones.* (Proverbs 3:7-8). By putting God first and seeking His kingdom, we lift our spirits to a new level of joy. The finest foods and supplements and the most prodigious amounts of exercising will go for naught unless we seek first the kingdom of God. This includes thinking of ourselves as God made us—whole and healthy—and recognizing the life force within us, which wants only wholeness and health. When this desire for health is firmly established in our minds and is followed up with positive deeds (eating properly and exercising regularly), it will result in our deliverance from any ill health. We can make a formula out of it: *A desire plus a deed will yield deliverance.* If we do our share, God will certainly do His! You believe that, don't you?

We can see that to have strong bones we must look once again to the whole spectrum of life—Spirit, soul, and body. We nourish the physical needs of the temple through nutrition and exercise. We nourish the spiritual needs through our awareness of our oneness with the mighty Architect who designed our temples.

When we seek first the kingdom, we will be led to true health. Our body temples will be beautiful and sturdy, our hearts shining with love, and our words sweet and joyful. And that will be a benefit too, for in Proverbs 16:24 we read: *Pleasant words are like a honeycomb, sweetness to the soul and health to the body.*

Your Perfect Prostate

We were created in the image of God, perfect and complete in every way. When we were given the incredible gift of life, we were, at the same time, given the means of sustaining and preserving that life. We were not programmed for physical failure, nor were we programmed for malfunctioning after reaching a certain chronological age. There is no God-given mechanism that ticks away the moments of our lives until it reaches "self-destruct." Our bodies, because they were created by God as His highest means of physical expression—the very dwelling places of His Holy Spirit—were designed to remain whole and perfect. It is the will of God.

Too often we fall victim to race beliefs which permeate our society. We come to accept the false idea that, because we are a certain age, certain things are going to "go wrong" in the body. Of course they will, if that is what we expect! But they do not have to and, what is more important, they should not, if we believe the teachings of Jesus Christ.

Charles Fillmore challenged us by exclaiming that we can be an Adam or a Christ or anything in between. It is entirely up to us. Each of us will become exactly what he believes himself to be—no more, no less. We are part of God, one with Him, but we will only manifest our God perfection to the degree that we are aware of Him. If we have limited physical bodies, we have a limited awareness of God.

We can change this, however. There is always the drive, the unceasing push, of the life force within us, seeking more and better life. It cannot help itself; that is its nature. The eternal, unchanging, perfect aspect of us longs for expression. It knows nothing of our foibles and race beliefs. How absurd to imagine that the Divinity within us could envision itself as weak or ill or imperfect in any way.

It is not your God nature which says that, because you have walked upon this planet for four or five decades, you can expect problems with your prostate gland. Isn't that nonsensical! And yet, that is what millions of men are programming into their obedient and ever-alert subconscious minds. We program it by repeating the idea over and over, living in fear of the "inevitability" of prostate (or any disease) symptoms until finally our prayers are answered and, like Job, we can anguish that: " . . . *the thing that I fear comes upon me, and what I dread befalls me.*" (Job 3:25)

Perhaps the use of the word prayers in this context surprised or shocked you. But the fact is that our *true* beliefs are those ideas that are continually dominant in our minds, and they will out-picture themselves in the words we habitually speak and in the deeds we routinely act out. These are our *true* prayers, far greater in power and effectiveness than a few minutes of spiritual endeavor that we formally call prayer. Emerson said our *every* act and *every* word is a prayer—one's entire life is a prayer, because it bespeaks the true feelings and beliefs of the heart.

This is a most important concept, because it opens the way for our realization that we are in complete charge of our lives. It brings us back to our original suggestion from Mr. Fillmore that we can be an Adam or a Christ. The choice is ours.

Mr. Fillmore also pronounced that *God fixes the plan of the structure and gives into the hands of man all the materials for building.* There are several "materials" that God provides us in our work of building the structure—the divine body temple. The first implement of construction is

the right use of our spiritual powers. We seek first our oneness with God, the source of all healing and life. We can
best do this through regular periods of meditation and
prayer. When we become still, we can hear the voice of the
Almighty as it speaks through us. We feel the thrill of the life
force as it brings wholeness to every cell, every gland of the
body. *When the mind is lifted up in meditation and prayer
the whole body glows with spiritual light,* Charles Fillmore
tells us. We can experience this for ourselves when we tune
into that divine center that lies at the core of our beings.

It is here, in the silence, that we systematically go about
our work of erasing the negative ideas of race consciousness
from our minds, establishing instead ideas of Truth—ideas
of perfection of the body temple. It is here, in the silence,
that we experience the dawn of a new awareness: *I am a
perfect expression of the divine Creator, who indwells every
atom of my body. I want to—I must—discover how I can let
that Divinity express with even greater beauty and greater
wholeness. It is my solemn duty to the Lord of my being.*

Therefore, we are led to do the things that will restore
us to perfection. We seek always for the stepping-stones to
lead us to our total good, which includes vibrant health of
every part of the body.

A Major Stepping-Stone

Perfect health is total physical success. To correct any
specific condition, such as prostatitis (or any disease), we
must correct the chemistry of the *whole* body. This means
that we must embark on a program of complete nutrition
that will nourish and regenerate the entire body.

Good nutrition begins with good protein. (See chapter
two, page 17, for listing of top-grade protein foods.)

Constructive carbohydrates are important because

245

they provide us with the proper fuels. Junk foods are poison to the prostate (and, indeed, the entire body); therefore, all destructive carbohydrates should be avoided. Constructive carbohydrates that are kind to the body are fresh fruits, fresh vegetables, and whole grains (including wholegrain breads). If a sweetener is desired, use small amounts of honey, blackstrap molasses, sorghum, or pure maple syrup. Sugar and white flour have no place in the body temple and can only defile it. And so can the delicious but dreadful "goodies" made from them. Include a constructive carbohydrate in every meal.

While fresh fruits are excellent carbohydrates and should be eaten regularly, citrus fruits may not be a good choice for someone with a prostate problem. They can be too caustic to the delicate tissues, and may be better left alone until improvement is shown.

In order to be complete, a meal should contain a small amount of unsaturated oil. A daily total of one or two teaspoonsful of raw, cold-pressed vegetable oil is recommended. If part of that quota can be cod liver oil, wheat germ oil, or pumpkin seed oil, the prostate will receive extra benefits. (These are available in capsule form if the liquid is unappealing to you.) We can use oils on vegetables, salads, toast, and in blender drinks. Raw, unsalted nuts and seeds also supply us with good oils, as well as high amounts of trace minerals.

Pitfalls

Special attention should be given to a particularly harmful group of "foods." Coffee is a major offender to the prostate. Decaffeinated coffee is no easier on the prostate, because the aromatic oils, rather than the caffeine, cause the trouble. Dr. John K. Lattimer, professor and chairman of the department of urology, College of Physicians and Surgeons of Columbia University, is an international authority on the prostate. He had this to say: *Once the prostate becomes slightly enlarged or slightly irritated, it becomes very susceptible to the effect of . . . coffee, . . . tea, any peppery [spicy] foods or alcohol. Thus, no matter what the cause of your prostate trouble, it will be somewhat improved by abstaining from these.*

Coffee, tea, spices, and alcohol should not be used by anyone who wants to protect the prostate. But why limit it to that? Coffee, tea, spices, and alcohol should not be used by *anyone* who wants to protect his health! In fact, they will not be used once we come to the realization that this is God's body, not ours. At that point, it becomes very easy to want to provide the life force with the best possible building materials.

There are other nutritional stepping-stones to prostate health. Perhaps you should be taking a high-potency multiple vitamin-mineral supplement each day. This supplement will contain all the vitamins, including all eleven of the B complex vitamins, as well as some important minerals. This is fine. But it may not be enough.

There are special considerations that have particular significance to the prostate gland. Vitamin A is necessary for the integrity of the epithelial tissues which line the gland. These tissues are our first line of defense against bacterial invasion, so they must be kept strong. Vitamin A can help in this. Cod liver oil is an excellent source of this vitamin. (It is also a wonderful, although not in taste, unsaturated oil.)

Vitamin C is also of great value. There is overwhelming evidence that adequate amounts help protect us from infection. Many scientists say that adequate amounts are between 1,000 and 5,000, and some say even up to 10,000 milligrams daily. Vitamin C is so valuable that once you determine your level, you will want to stay with it always.

In case of prostate infection, there is a wonder-working little drink that might be of help. In a glass of water, dissolve one teaspoonful of vitamin C powder and one teaspoonful of liquid chlorophyll. Sip this throughout the day. When it is finished, another batch can be made and sipped on. The chlorophyll helps to buffer the acid in the vitamin C which for some people might result in temporary diarrhea when taken in such large amounts. (One teaspoonful of granular vitamin C contains about 5,000 milligrams.) Incidentally, this drink is good "first aid" for any infection, not just prostate.

Zinc is indicated as important to the prostate. In a long-term experiment reported to the American Medical Association meeting in 1974, men with prostate problems given zinc supplements daily reported a reduction in symptoms, and more than seventy percent reported actual shrinkage of enlarged prostates. It seems that taking extra zinc could be wise.

Also wise could be the use of lecithin. One or more tablespoonsful of lecithin granules can help keep the tiny blood vessels clear, thereby better enabling the blood containing the vital nutrients to reach the prostate cells. Lecithin granules can be sprinkled on salads, soups, and vegetables, and put into blender drinks. It is a good adjunct to a proper diet.

Pumpkins Not Just for Halloween

The benefits of taking pumpkin seed oil have already been mentioned. There is a factor in pumpkin seeds that is very helpful to the prostate. In addition to taking the oil (liquid or capsules), we can also eat the pumpkin seeds. They are a delicious and healthful snack. Raw, unsalted pumpkin seeds can be purchased already hulled at most health food stores. Nibble away to your heart's (and prostate's) content!

Beverages and Baths

There are still further stepping-stones. Mildly diuretic herbal teas can be used. Varieties such as uva ursi, shave grass, watermelon seed, and bucchu are good. Each has a unique flavor, so you will have to choose the ones you like best.

Another benefit to the prostate is a warm bath. Just sitting in a warm bath tends to relax the muscles and open the blood vessels and small ducts. The more they open, the more opportunity there is for foreign matter to break free and to be flushed out. In this age of quick showers, the beneficial effects of the warm bath should not be overlooked.

A Final Step

We come now to one more stepping-stone, a very major one: Exercise. Mild physical exercise is most invigorating to the organs and glands in the pelvic region. Walking is especially good, and it pays extra dividends in cardio-vascular health. Try to take a brisk walk every day.

Since gravity is always pulling our glands and organs downward, squeezing and constricting them, it is very beneficial to reverse this gravitational pull. An easy way to do this is to spend about fifteen minutes a day on a slantboard. With the feet raised in this manner, the blood can circulate more freely into those areas that are usually constricted by gravity. If you are going to use a slantboard, however, be sure to begin by lying on it for only a minute or two. Then gradually increase the time. When you want to get up, do it very slowly, allowing the body to become re-accustomed to the upright position. *Do not stand up right away!*

Pearl of Great Price

We have now seen several very useful stepping-stones that can lead to a healthy prostate. The first was meditation and prayer. When we begin with that step, the others become easier. Putting God first puts all else into proper perspective. We begin to see that we are capable of perfection—the perfection of the Almighty. Then the various subsequent stepping-stones come more clearly into view.

All challenges submit to the healing power of the life force if given the opportunity. We provide the life force with that opportunity when we obey the physical laws of nutrition and exercise that God ordained as the means by which the body temple is to be constructed.

A healthy prostate is the fruit of a healthy body. When the spiritual, mental, and physical laws are obeyed, race beliefs have no power in our lives. We desire perfection, and we take the proper steps to achieve it. Solid health becomes ours and, once we have it, we realize it was worth the effort. It is our natural state and, because it is the Father's will for us, it becomes the pearl of great price.

Youthfulness Is Yours

Leroy "Satchel" Paige never knew how old he was. He never had a birth certificate nor was there anyone who could tell him his age. From the time he pitched in the old "Negro League" to the time when racial barriers were removed and he broke into the major leagues as a (some thought fifty-year-old) "rookie," he could not be sure of his age. When asked how old he was, Satchel Paige would answer, "How old would you be if you did not know how old you were?"

What a wonderful answer to such a meaningless question. A subtle challenge is offered by it. Ask it of yourself. How old would you be if you did not know how old you are?

If you ponder the question for a few minutes, you will discover two things. The first is the absurdity of counting years as an identification of a person. And the second is that it is we who decide how old we really are!

Time Is Not Toxic

What does age indicate? It merely tells us how many times we have been around the sun since exiting the womb. Should our age have any significance to our health? Certainly not! Time is not toxic. Age is chronological, not pathological. The great surgeon Dr. Hans Selye once said, "In all of my autopsies (and I have performed quite a few), I have never seen a man who died of old age." There is nothing disease-causing about age or time. Age does not decay bodies. The truth is that age can strengthen bodies. Age will strengthen bodies that are growing toward perfection. Think of that! As we work on improving our bodies, time becomes our ally because it gives us a period, a duration, to improve ourselves. And that which is constantly improved cannot perish.

It is not time that does us harm but our *belief* in the power of time to harm us. And therein lies one of the keys to perpetual youthfulness. Jesus said: . . . *"According to your faith be it done to you."* (Matt. 9:29) If it is our belief that time has some magical power to harm us, then according to our faith it will be done to us. Ultimately our bodies are obedient to our minds. Our bodies are mirrors of what our minds believe. If our minds firmly believe that we should live to be only threescore and ten, then we will most assuredly find a way to die at age seventy.

It has been said that we are all tattooed in our cradles with the belief of our tribe. All our lives we have been told by our parents and friends, and we have seen in the movies and on television, that certain birthdays have special significance. When we have gone around the sun twenty-one times, we are adults. When we have gone around the sun thirty-five times, we have "tired blood." Having completed forty revolutions, we are now entering "middle age." And after sixty-five turns around the sun, we must retire from life and await the grim reaper! Our lives are broken into periods, and every period finds us getting older. Our subconscious minds accept this fact and proceed to manifest this belief in our bodies. We cannot be anything different from what we believe ourselves to be.

Unity author Mary Katherine MacDougall says: *Most of us need to stop thinking about old age, our own and that of others. It is too easy to place someone in an age category, thinking that at any given age he can do only certain things.*

We are likely to pigeonhole people by ages.

Think Youth, Speak Youth

The first area of change must be in our minds. We can, through the use of denials and affirmations, change our attitudes toward aging. By changing our subconscious minds, we will change our attitudes. When our attitudes change, our life-styles will change. When our life-styles change, our lives change.

Our minds are encrusted with years of belief in aging and death. In order to dissolve these false impressions, we must deny that time has power over us. We should repeat many times each day: *Time has no power over me; it cannot hurt me.*

Next, we must affirm what is true about our bodies: The life force within us knows nothing about disease, decay, or death. It knows only life, and it seeks only life. It is we who, with our negative thoughts and harmful deeds, inhibit the life force from fully expressing itself. The only way we can assist the life force is by allowing it to unfold through us. We should affirm daily: *I allow the life force within me to express completely.*

Russell Kemp in his book *Live Youthfully Now* says: *Your body, which is always the obedient mirror of your mind, will outwardly display the youth you are affirming as soon as your subconscious acceptance of it is complete.*

Catherine Ponder offers a marvelous method of working with the faculty of life. She says: *The best method of activating the mighty life force within you is this: in your quiet times of relaxation and rest, start at the top of the head and mentally go down through the various parts of the body, decreeing "LIFE, LIFE, LIFE." As you decree it, you will feel a certain current of excitement, enthusiasm, and a warm electrical energy come alive within you in various parts of the body.*

Charles Fillmore also had something germane to say about this subject: *The vital energy of eternal life exists in every cell of our body. Science proclaims that . . . man's body would live forever if it were not for his brain.* In other words, if we were to allow the universal life force, which is in each of us, to *fully* express, instead of allowing our race beliefs to dictate to us, there would be no aging. On another occasion, he said: *God did not create man to die; death is a result of a transgression of law. Christianity teaches that man was created to live in his body, refining it as his thoughts unfold, and that the work of the Christ . . . is to unite Spirit, soul, and body here on earth . . . every thought of death, or the possibility of leaving the body, must be put out of the mind.*

Begin to see yourself as a vibrant, whole, and healthy member of a universe that knows and seeks only life. "Plug into" your divine inheritance. Allow the life force within you to manifest in its fullness, unencumbered by race beliefs.

As we begin to change our thought patterns to ideas of health and wholeness, we will also begin seeking a way of life to complement this new mental attitude. This, of course, requires changing our eating habits. Charles Fillmore said: *We should spiritualize our thoughts and refine the food we eat to correspond.*

We all know that there are definite laws governing the body temple. It is incumbent upon everyone desiring to beautify and preserve this temple to learn what the body needs and to present it with the finest raw materials available.

Eating for Youthfulness

Any talk of rebuilding, renewing, and preserving the body temple must begin with protein. Protein, the proper kinds in the proper amounts, is the *only* means the body has of building new tissues. Without a sufficient amount of protein the human body cannot maintain nor renew itself.

We could commission the finest architect to design the most magnificent temple and then hire the best contractor to build the structure; however, if we did not have bricks and mortar, the beautiful temple could not be built and would exist only in its potential.

The divine Architect has designed perfection into each one of our one hundred trillion cells. Within each cell dwells a master Builder ready to translate that blueprint into flesh and blood fact. But it needs raw materials to do so. Top-grade protein provides the bricks and mortar that God uses to build tissue. Without it, our physical perfection exists only in potential. Therefore, the first nutritional consideration must be protein. (See your specially marked section in chapter two, page 17.)

The next consideration is to give our bodies some good carbohydrate at every meal. Carbohydrates act as a fuel which, in addition to sparing the precious protein to allow it to renew us, gives us the energy of metabolism to keep our miracle machines running effortlessly.

It is in the area of carbohydrate ingestion that we make the biggest nutritional mistake. It is the eating of destructive carbohydrates, especially sugar and white flour, that contributes more to physiological deterioration than any other single nutritional cause. We must choose our carbohydrates carefully, being sure to put the finest fuel into our bodies.

All machines need oil. The miracle machine that is our body is no exception. However, for maximum performance, we must choose our oils carefully. Oils from animal sources, in the form of fat, are to be shunned. They are highly saturated, and the body has trouble handling them in large amounts.

The best oils are raw, unhydrogenated vegetable oils containing no preservatives. Some good, tasty oils are safflower oil, corn oil, sunflower seed oil, and sesame seed oil. These are best eaten raw on salads or vegetables and can even be used in soups.

Two oils that have a special application in a program of rejuvenation are cod liver oil and wheat germ oil. Neither has a taste that lends itself to cooking or mixing with food (although wheat germ oil can be put into a blender drink and will not be tasted). However, they are such marvelous oils that it may behoove us to include them in our nutrition regime.

Cod liver oil is rich in vitamins A and D. Vitamin A is needed for healthy skin and eyes, and vitamin D is essential for strong bones.

Wheat germ oil, on the other hand, is most noted for its ability to increase stamina and provide some of the raw materials for the manufacture of testosterone and estrogen, the male and female sex hormones. It is a highly concentrated food, since it requires about five pounds of wheat to make one teaspoonful of the oil! Both cod liver oil and wheat germ oil are available in capsule form.

Other sources of oils are nuts and seeds. These foods make fine snacks, and they should be eaten only raw and unsalted.

Special Supplements

Certain vitamins and minerals are especially suited to a program of youthful longevity. However, the primary supplement should be in the form of a multiple vitamin-mineral tablet with an adequate amount of all the essentials, including strong amounts of the complete (all eleven) B complex. This is your insurance. It will assure at least a minimum amount of the needed vitamins and minerals.

We know that the process we call aging begins with our subconscious minds' belief in it. After the subconscious embraces this belief, however, it filters into our lives, finally manifesting in our bodies as a physiological fact.

Among the theories of aging, the most popular shows it to be caused by the formation of harmful peroxides in the body. These are caused when oxygen interacts with polyunsaturates in the body tissues. Both are essential to our existence, but when the interaction is not controlled, the proteins in our bodies are harmed and a process we call aging occurs.

Vitamin C and vitamin E are very powerful antioxidants. In other words, they can help to control the unwanted interaction between oxygen and the polyunsaturates. Roger J. Williams, one of America's greatest biochemists, writes: *Ascorbic acid (vitamin C) may delay old age because it has strong antioxidant properties (prevents unwanted oxidation). . . . Vitamin E is thought to be the leading agent for the prevention of peroxidation. . . . As a practical matter, providing plenty of vitamin E and ascorbic acid, both harmless antioxidants, is indicated as a possible means of preventing premature aging. . . .*

Dr. Linus Pauling, two-time winner of the Nobel prize, agrees wholeheartedly. He writes: *Vitamin E is the principal fat-soluble antioxidant, and vitamin C (ascorbic acid) is the principal water-soluble antioxidant. They probably cooperate in providing protection for our bodies and slowing the aging process.*

How much should we take of these wonderful vitamins

if we feel we need them? Dr. Pauling's suggestion concerning vitamin E is that: *A younger person might do well on 100 I.U. per day, an older one on 400 I.U. or 800 I.U.*

As far as vitamin C is concerned, he suggests that . . . *for the best of health . . . an intake of between 1 g and 5 g (1,000 milligrams and 5,000 milligrams) per day is needed by most people. An even larger intake may confer additional benefit. I take 10 g (10,000 milligrams) per day. In addition, the intake of sugar should be kept low, and some other vitamins should be taken — vitamin E, vitamin A, and the B vitamins.*

If, after reading what these famous scientists have to say about supplements, you decide you would like to try them, remember that good nutrition begins with good food, not with vitamin and mineral supplements. First, be sure your diet is optimum, and then add any vitamins and minerals you feel you need.

Young Bodies Move

It is not within the purview of this book to deal at length with exercise. There are wonderful books that deal quite extensively with the subject. The important point to be made is that a regime of regular exercise is essential if any progress is to be made in restoring and renewing health to the body.

By regular exercise we mean engaging in an activity that coaxes (not forces) the body to approach its present physical limits. Because each of us has a unique individuality, because we all begin to rehabilitate ourselves on different levels, this exercise might be a walk around the block for one person or a jog of ten miles for another.

While this chapter was being written, the following article appeared in a news magazine: *"People don't die of old age, they die of neglect. I work at being a superman,"* pro-

claimed Jack La Lanne. The body builder kept his image afloat for his 65th birthday by swimming over a mile with his feet in shackles, towing 65 boats laden with 6,500 pounds of wood pulp. . . . Says the body builder: "I'm going to live to be at least 150." It obviously takes a great deal of exercise to challenge Mr. La Lanne's body. But that is because he has worked to develop it. (As a child, Jack La Lanne was puny and sickly, until he decided that there was something he could do about it.)

Choose an exercise that appeals to you. A long, brisk walk is great, as are jogging, swimming, rope jumping, yoga, cycling, and many others. Remember to regularly coax your body to approach its present limits.

To rejuvenate our bodies, we must first rejuvenate our minds. Our subconscious must embrace the idea that time is not toxic. Time cannot harm us. We are timeless creatures existing in the continuum of God's love. Our bodies will ultimately manifest what our minds think we are. We can be nothing more. When we rid ourselves of the consciousness of age, our bodies will want to renew themselves. When we realize that we are truly temples of God, it will be our most fervent desire to renew and rejuvenate our temples.

We know too that we can only function within the self-imposed boundaries of our present consciousness. If, in our present consciousness, we need food and drink in order to live, then we had better eat the most nourishing foods and drink the finest beverages if we want to have beautiful body temples. If our desire is perfect health, then our deeds must follow, for a desire without a deed is a dead end.

Man can grow qualitatively without limit. This makes us potentially invincible because what is constantly improved cannot perish.

The cells of our bodies are always renewing themselves. As long as our thoughts are coming from our Christ

259

center and we are following the physical laws of body renewal, we must never think of how old we are. Our
thoughts instead should be of how *new* we are.

We must never begin a sentence with "At my
age. . . . " We should follow the advice of the man who,
when asked his age, replied, "My age is none of *my* business."

And lastly, we should never decide how long we want
to live. That too is none of our business. Because our
parents and grandparents lived to be seventy-two does not
mean that this fact should limit us. Why should we say, "I'll
live to be seventy-two," or "ninety," or even "150"? Why
limit ourselves? Why let our good get in the way of our better? If we put our lives in the hands of God, why not put our
total lives in the hands of God? Why program our own
deaths?

Our lives are not just ephemeral manifestations in an
epic universal struggle of life and death. We have no beginning, and we have no end. We are ageless creations of a
timeless Creator.

Our test then is simple, but it is not easy. It is to seek
first the kingdom of God and to obey *all* of the laws that
God has set forth. When we do this, when we put God first
in our lives and obey His laws, we will begin manifesting the
greatest promise of the Scriptures. Instead of fearing an end
that is without life, we will demonstrate a life that is without
end.

Decision for Vision

. . . the blind men came to him; and Jesus said to them, "Do you believe that I am able to do this?" They said to him, "Yes, Lord." Then he touched their eyes, saying, "According to your faith be it done to you." And their eyes were opened. (Matt. 9:28-30)

What do you believe about *your* eyes, those great windows of the soul through which peers the eternal One? Like miniature searchlights our eyes scan the heavens and the Earth, questioning, seeking, identifying the other parts of creation from which they, themselves, are inseparable.

In view of the fact that life is ever new—billions of cells being born each second, and this includes eye cells—there is absolutely no need to accept the race belief that the body wears out. There is no need to accept the false notion that eyes must grow dim as years add up. We can lift our beliefs and thoughts to the Truth, just as the psalmist who sang: *I lift up my eyes to the hills.* (Psalms 121:1)

We instinctively seem to recognize that there is something special about our eyes. They are more than just another part of our anatomy. They represent a link between our outer world and our soul. They are symbolic of that inner sight which illumines our path and "sees" the Truth. This is what Jesus Christ meant when He said: *". . . blessed are your eyes, for they see . . . ."* (Matt. 13:16)

Have you ever noticed that an animal will look you in the eyes? Why is that? Why doesn't it look at your shoulder or your knee? There is something even in animals which seems to know that we communicate through our eyes— that they are special. When we say to another that we see the Christ in him, we look into his eyes, don't we? What marvelous instruments the eyes are, that even the animals recognize their singularity.

Myrtle Fillmore had some pertinent words to say about the eyes: *The eyes are the physical organs that are the out-picturing of the capacity of the mind to discern, mentally, physically, spiritually, all that is. Seeing is a mental process; and the eyes are the instruments that register what the mind has been trained to think and to behold. When our mental processes are in perfectly harmonious accord with the ideas of Divine Mind, our sight is perfect and our eyes function properly . . . .*

Let's look (notice how we continually use terms of vision to refer to our understanding and insight!) at some of the inner meanings behind the outer problems of the eyes. And keep in mind how often we use these vision terms. Try to see (oops, there's another one!) how often you employ such words as "see" or "look at" or "notice." It might surprise you.

The condition of our eyes depends on two things: the way we look at things specifically, and our mental viewpoint generally. We have to check on ourselves to determine how we are "looking at" life. Eye problems force us to analyze how we are mentally viewing our world.

It has been said that eye trouble means "I" trouble. In other words, problems in the eyes are reflecting problems in our egos or our personalities—what we are thinking and feeling.

There are some fascinating *metaphysical interpretations* to various eye conditions. Inflamed eyeballs, for instance, might mean that one is "seeing red" about some particular situation in his life.

Cataracts can often reflect a mind which is closed to things or even closed to the fact that some influence could be trying to "pull the wool over the eyes." This condition is possibly a result of not wanting to look at things clearly or face them head-on.

Glaucoma may represent a rigid resistance to all attempts at changing one's point of view. The eyeball becomes as inflexible as the opinions one holds regarding others' behavior.

Myopia could represent one's refusal to see things in the proper way, and so shortsightedness results.

Remember, these are *metaphysical* interpretations only.

Once you begin analyzing and identifying what the physical manifestation is, it becomes easy to analyze and identify the corresponding inner conditions which may have caused it all. And once this is done, you can then take steps to change those inner conditions.

Develop Inner Vision

Persistent use of your faculty of imagination is one of the best and quickest means of overcoming any vision problems. During your daily meditation periods, close your eyes and feel the warmth of God's healing activity flowing to and through your eyes. Think of your eyes as brightly beaming beacons, filled with power and ability to see all.

It is sometimes helpful to picture a healing scene. *And Jesus in pity touched their eyes, and immediately they received their sight and followed him.* (Matt. 20:34) Perhaps it appeals to you to picture and feel the hands of Jesus Christ upon your eyes, blessing and restoring them. Whatever healing image is comfortable to you will, if used with belief and joy and thanksgiving, be beneficial.

Notice the ending to the above Scripture passage: [they] *followed him*. This is important because there can be no *permanent* healing without a change in consciousness—a change in the way we think and feel. We must *follow him*. We must live from our Christ consciousness, and this means that in all things we seek first the kingdom. It also means that we will be loving to all people at all times and in all situations.

Once you have established the metaphysical causes of your eye condition and have begun to work on clearing them out, there is other work to be done as well. The eyes, as a part of the physical body temple, need nourishment. They must be thoughtfully and lovingly fed.

Feeding the Eyes

In all cases, the body (including eyes) requires certain raw materials. These include adequate protein (especially at breakfast). (See chapter two, page 17, for complete listing.)

The body also requires constructive carbohydrates. These are in fresh fruits, fresh vegetables, and whole grains. This list of constructive carbohydrates may seem short, but when one considers the plethora of fruits, vegetables, and whole grains (including whole-grain baked goods, cereals, etc.) available, the number of wholesome carbohydrates expands dramatically.

The list of destructive carbohydrates is almost endless. The most insidious offenders are sugar, white flour, cola drinks, and junk foods of any kind.

Required also is some good form of oil each day. Excellent oils are raw and unprocessed vegetable oils, such as safflower, sunflower, corn, soy, and sesame. Wheat germ oil also is good. Cod liver oil has very special significance for the health of the eyes because of its high content of natural vitamin A.

After making sure that your diet is as healthful as possible, you can then add certain supplements which will help the eyes. A strong multiple vitamin is the best place to begin your supplementation. Next you may want to add some extra vitamin A and a complete (all eleven of the B vitamins) B complex. Vitamin C is required in extra amounts and a C complex is often helpful. The C complex is a tablet which contains, in addition to vitamin C, bioflavonoids and rutin. A good multiple mineral supplement is also worthwhile and will round out your program.

In the case of cataract it may be beneficial to add extra amounts of vitamin B2 (riboflavin) and vitamin E.

Remember that total wholeness requires total nutrition—proper diet along with proper supplementation. There is no magic pill for overcoming a vision problem. Work in the nutrition area requires the same dedication and completeness as does work in mental areas.

Exercise the Eyes

No campaign toward wholeness, even of the eyes, is complete without some form of exercise. Traditional body movement, such as *brisk* walking, jogging, yoga, calisthenics, bicycling, square dancing, and certain sports are excellent for improving the general condition of the body. Most importantly, they improve circulation, which is the body's only means of bringing nourishment to the eyes. In order to obtain maximum results from exercises, they must be done cheerfully and *regularly*.

But there are also specific exercises designed solely for the eyes and which are extremely helpful. There are numerous books available that can provide detailed information on eye exercises. The Bates method has been a popular source of help and is highly recommended. There are others. Make a point of incorporating some eye exercises into your daily self-help program. The investment of a few moments a day can pay big dividends in vision improvement.

Always remember to keep the eyes rested and relaxed. When doing close-up work, take frequent breaks of looking at a distance. And vice versa.

"Looking" for Improvement

It seems to be commonly accepted that the eyes reflect the soul. Fear, anger, and resentment can be seen in someone's eyes—they take on a "hard" look. On the other hand, seeing only the beauty in life and looking toward God make the eyes shine and soften in appearance. And this seems only natural, doesn't it?

If you have a problem with your eyes and you really want to overcome it, don't condemn your eyes or eyeglasses. Whenever you think of your eyes, bless them. This correction of attitude is a good place to start in correcting the eyes.

Also, never discuss poor eyesight or whatever the condition happens to be. Never say things like, "I'm as blind as a bat without my glasses!" There is very little healing power available to anyone who affirms a false condition to himself or to others. If you speak about your condition, you are in effect claiming it for yourself.

The eyes, like any other part of the body, respond to your thoughts and words. Praise them. Bless them. Encourage them. Image them as perfect. Nourish them properly. Exercise them regularly, and you will soon be "seeing" good results.

266

Ears to Hear

"Incline your ear, and come to me; hear, that your soul may live; and I will make with you an everlasting covenant . . . . " (Isa. 55:3)

What a miracle of perfection is the human ear! Have you ever seen the tiny ear of a newborn baby? It is like a small seashell, perfectly sculptured in every detail. Even a developing fetus exhibits the miniature seashell structures which are to become fully-fashioned human ears. They are one of the wonders of the body temple.

And yet, something deep within us seems to know that the ears are much more than physical protuberances on the sides of our heads. Something tells us that hearing is much more than receiving sound waves. While it is true that the ears relay sound impressions to the brain, this is only the beginning. The brain must interpret the sounds and then make judgments based upon these interpretations. The ear is therefore more than a physical organ; it represents the listening mind or Spirit. *"He who has ears to hear, let him hear,"* (Matt. 11:15) were Jesus' words. He meant that although we may take in sounds—words—we sometimes do not really *hear* the message. . . . *having ears, do you not hear?* (Mark 8:18) He asked. Are we always tuned in to universal Mind? Do we hear the promptings of the Christ within?

Ears are wonderful things. They help coordinate the sounds of the outer world with the sounds of our inner world. The inner part of our ear actually has two openings:

one that leads to the outside and one that leads inward. Perhaps this is symbolic of the role hearing plays in our lives.

Inner Listening

How many times have you heard a person who is hard-of-hearing say, "I can hear what I want to hear"? There is a selective listening technique that we all possess. We often seem to be able to hear the things that we really want to hear. We can use this ability in a positive and constructive way by allowing only the positive and constructive sounds to become part of our minds.

We should make a practice of screening sounds, letting only the harmonious ones enter the inner sanctity of our being. Our outer world can sound very chaotic and harsh and negative to us if we let it. Instead, let us listen only for the good—the godly. There is much beautiful and loving sound around us if we tune in to it.

But we should also cultivate an inner listening. It is only when we turn our ears inward that we hear that *still, small voice* which speaks to us in the peaceful recesses of our souls. This is the highest form of listening. It is where we receive guidance, wisdom, answers, and comfort.

Many people throughout history have "heard" voices speaking within them. The Bible recounts several such cases and, of course, one cannot forget the case of Joan of Arc. History was often changed through the direction of these inner voices.

And it is not only history that has been affected. The arts also owe some of their finest creations to inner sounds. Beethoven was virtually deaf when he wrote some of his most inspiring music. He "heard" the great melodies and harmonies with his inner ear. But he is not the only one.

Music always comes from within the soul of the composer. It is clearly heard within before a note of it is ever put on paper or played on an instrument.

The point is that if we are interested in lifting our consciousness and living creatively, we will have to develop our inner listening.

Now Hear This

Metaphysicians have come up with some interesting and logical explanations of ear problems. An earache, for example, may suggest some painful incident (or words) which is not clearly understood. So the ear responds by hurting. Sometimes an earache can develop because we are hearing something we cannot accept.

We saw a perfect example of this in a close friend of ours. When he first discovered Unity, he was hungry to learn more of the teachings. He went immediately to a six-day retreat at Unity Village, at which he saturated himself with words of Truth. During the retreat, he suddenly developed a very painful earache which forced him to miss a day of activities. He could not understand it because he rarely gets ill. As soon as the retreat was over and he left for home, the earache disappeared.

Our friend later realized that the earache was a result of his trying to hear too much Truth—too much that was contrary to his former beliefs—at one time. It became too painful and was more than he could handle. There is no doubt in our friend's mind that this was the primary cause of the earache!

Loss of hearing can also be attributed to a desire to shut out things that are not pleasant or comfortable. Over the years a person can gradually become deaf to his spouse. Once you start looking for the meanings behind the physical symptoms, it becomes quite easy to discover them. This is good practice for ourselves, but you can see how wrong it would be to do it with others. As Vera Dawson Tait has remarked: *Let's mind our own spiritual business!*

Silence, Please

Our ears enable us to hear the Word! With them we hear teachings of the Master through the voices of our ministers and instructors. And this is good.

We should also have a daily period of quiet time in which we listen to the silence within. This is a time of perfect peace—of meditation. This is our special time.

Charles Fillmore discusses "Spiritual Hearing" in *Teach Us to Pray: Practice giving ear or listening with your mind to the Lord. You will acquire the ability to make contact with the mind radiations of Christ and concentrate them in your mind and actually hear His voice.*

It is during these quiet times that you can do much work on your wonderful ears. After listening within, take several moments to focus your efforts on your ears. Praise them and encourage them to hear God's delightful sounds. The tremendous power of imagination can be helpful in this respect. Take time to give attention to your ears.

The body is like a child. It needs constant prompting and training and discipline and praise and appreciation. Your body needs your attention, your love, your training. This instruction comes to us from Myrtle Fillmore's valuable book *How to Let God Help You.*

We must spiritually nourish our ears as Mrs. Fillmore suggests. They love it and will gratefully respond.

Foods for Hearing

There is also physical nourishment to be considered. The ears, like any part of the physical body, require proper nutrients.

If you desire good health (and this includes good hearing), ask yourself the following questions:

Am I eating a good breakfast? (A cup of coffee and a doughnut do *not* constitute a good breakfast!) A good breakfast contains adequate protein and a suitable carbohydrate. Eggs and toast make up the traditional breakfast, and the combination is a wonderful choice (if the toast is made with whole-grain bread and Better Butter is used). But one does not have to eat eggs in the morning in order to be well nourished. Many people prefer cereal in the morning. Of course, the devitalized popular cereals have no place in the body temple, but cereals such as oatmeal and the granola types with lots of nuts and seeds are acceptable, especially when served with milk to improve the protein quality. Some prefer cottage cheese and fresh fruit in the morning. Still others enjoy leftover chicken or turkey with an apple. There are no strict rules except to give your body adequate protein and a good carbohydrate.

Am I getting enough protein with my other meals? Remember, the need for protein does not end at breakfast.

Am I avoiding all "junk foods," which only serve to debase the body temple? (To make a list of these foods would be too long and tedious. Each of us knows in his heart-of-hearts just what junk foods are.)

Am I eating only the essential carbohydrates at each meal?

Have I eliminated caffeine, alcohol, tobacco, and sugar?

Am I supplying my precious ear tissues with adequate

271

vitamins and minerals each day? It is usually a good idea to take a strong, complete multiple vitamin-mineral tablet daily. Added to this may be extra amounts of vitamin A, a complete B complex, vitamin C, and extra minerals.

If you can honestly answer yes to all of these questions, you can relax in the knowledge that you are doing your share nutritionally. You are providing the life force with the proper raw materials with which it can maintain and improve your hearing ability. When you do your share, you can always have trust in the life force to do its share.

Feed your ears. Nourish them. Give them the nutrients they need and deserve.

Eat with the understanding that you are providing God-given materials which the inner intelligence will use to nourish and cleanse and renew all of your body every day. (Myrtle Fillmore in *How to Let God Help You.*)

Exercise for the Ears

Exercise my ears? Absolutely! All parts of the body require movement. The ears are no exception. A good idea is to move the lower jaw in and out about twenty times. Gently stretch it as far forward as you can. Also, pull as hard as you *comfortably* can on the earlobes. This helps circulation and loosens up wax deposits.

Of course the more traditional exercises are also important. Walking, swimming, yoga, calisthenics, aerobic dancing, and countless others help to strengthen the body in general, to circulate nutrients and to carry away the waste products of metabolism.

Let your body know the joy of your loving attention and interest; give it the exercise it needs. This admonition is from Myrtle Fillmore, and a good one it is.

A Final Hearing

So you see that there are many things you can do to improve and maintain your hearing. It is entirely up to you as to how much effort you want to make on behalf of your ears. The points to remember are:

1. Be aware that perfect hearing is God's will for you.

2. Use meditation and imaging daily.

3. Listen to only the sweet sounds—the harmonies around you.

4. Follow proper nutritional guidelines.

5. Get adequate regular exercise.

Train your ears to hear the harmony of the universe about you. Learn to listen for the loveliness. Screen your sounds. Shut out the negatives. Ask yourself, what am I listening to? If your answer is less than good, begin now to change your thinking and your feelings by allowing only the harmonious to enter your ears. Remind yourself frequently that: *I listen with love.*

And, finally, always remember to bless your ears. Bless them and give thanks for the hearing improvement that is now yours.

Don't Depend on Drugs

. . . "I am the bread of life; he who comes to me shall not hunger, and he who believes in me shall never thirst." (John 6:35)

Are you hungering and thirsting for something to satisfy an emptiness in your life? Have you chased down countless paths in search of a prize which, once captured, would fill a void within your soul and give meaning to your life? But one by one the prizes disappointed, the chase grew more frantic, the despair began to overwhelm. And, finally, on one gray day when it seemed as if the sun would never shine again, you reached for an artificial stimulant—a drug—perhaps a "socially acceptable" drug such as alcohol or a tranquilizer, or perhaps it was an illegal substance. And thus was born a habit which slowly grew into a curse.

By now you know deep down in your soul that answers do not lie in pills, powders, or liquids. The search for meaning in our lives can never be satisfied with outside things. There is no antidote for emptiness and feelings of futility that can be swallowed, injected, or inhaled.

A life so meaningless that it has to be "escaped" is a life that has not yet discovered its own divinity and oneness with the universe. And those who try to escape life carry their confinement on their backs.

If you have been running away from your own existence and are now weary of the race, take heart, for things can be different if you want them to be!

Jesus revealed that the kingdom of God is within. It is

within *you* and always has been. If this is so, the only way a person can be totally happy, fulfilled, and at peace is to *look within*. You have tried looking to the outer world for satisfaction, and you have discovered it is not there. Not knowing where to look further and not knowing that your search was really a search for God, you sank into despair and frustration, seeking temporary escape with artificial stimulants or hallucinogens.

And temporary they were because you found, when their effects wore off, nothing had changed. The same feelings, fears, and dissatisfactions reared their heads again, and so the cycle was repeated. What you must finally realize is that the only thing that can completely lift you out of the sense of emptiness and discontent that gnaws at you is the realization of who and what you really are: a spiritual being who has at his fingertips all the goodness of this marvelous universe.

No one can "give" you God, simply because God has never been taken away from you. God has always been with you, although you may not have realized it. And to *experience* the presence of the Creator in you is something you, and you alone, must do. But you can be guided toward the experience through reading and studying spiritual writings, attending classes and worship services, and, most importantly, through daily sessions of quiet prayer and meditation.

Become acquainted with the four Gospels, (Matthew, Mark, Luke, and John) and discover firsthand the profound teachings of Jesus Christ. Take His words and their meaning into your heart, and use them as a guide to make contact with that Power within, which will lift, strengthen, and sustain you. Realize that you are the maker of your own world and that everything in your life is an inestimable gift for your own growth. Become familiar with the love and guidance of God. Once you open yourself to God's love and guidance you will become more trusting.

Let your life become anchored in the truth of your existence, which is that it is not meaningless, empty, and at the mercy of things "out there." Change your consciousness from that of victim to that of victor, and you will triumph!

The Truth of the Matter

Psychology has long been attempting to explain drug addiction through frustration, yearning, deprivation, and even genetics. Through metaphysics we can fully understand the challenge.

The truth is that it is natural to yearn for the good things in life: happiness, success, love, and so on. In fact, these things are God's will for His children. They are gifts given to us freely, generously, and unconditionally. The power that a drug has over us is due merely to our false belief that the only way we can experience happiness is through "supplementing" God's gift by ingesting a pill or a powder or a liquid. But since God has held back nothing from His creations, this is to look without for something we already possess within.

Once you realize that God will never withhold anything good from His children, the dependency on drugs will cease. Drug addiction is actually a form of idolatry since it is a prayer to a material substance to supply what has already been supplied by God but not yet recognized by the individual. Drugs, in themselves, have no power to make you happy. The power is already within you. Drugs have *only* the power you give them.

Drugs can be broken down into three general types: stimulants—drugs that stimulate the central nervous system; depressants—drugs that depress the central nervous system; and hallucinogens—drugs that alter perceptions of reality. Abuse of these substances causes both physical and psychological damage.

Among the stimulants, amphetamines (street-named speed, uppers, pep pills, etc.) can cause convulsions, coma, and brain damage. Cocaine (coke, snow, white lady, toot, etc.) will cause damage to the nasal passages, sleeplessness, and anxiety. Nicotine (yes, nicotine is a drug and a stimulant!) has been closely linked with cancer and heart disease. All can easily create psychological dependencies.

Depressants are addictive. Among the popular depressants, barbiturates (downers, barbs, etc.) elicit a loss of appetite and very severe withdrawal symptoms. The same holds true with narcotics (morphine, heroin, Darvon, Percodan, codeine, etc.). Alcohol, one of the most popular depressant drugs, can wreak havoc in the body temple, especially the heart, liver, and brain cells. Like all depressants, it too is addictive. (This is especially true in teenagers who, because of differences in their body chemistry, can develop alcoholism much more rapidly than a mature adult!)

Hallucinogens are dangerous, not only because of what they do to the user but also because of what the user, in a state of altered perception, does to himself and to others. Marijuana and hashish (pot, grass, hash, etc.) cause damage to the lungs and reproductive system. PCP (angel dust) causes severe anxiety or depression and hallucination. LSD eventuates severe mood swings and emotional breakdown, as do mescaline and psilocybin (magic mushrooms).

It is rather obvious that the effects of these drugs are severe. But what about the effects of the more socially acceptable anti-anxiety drugs, the benzodiazepines, such as Valium, Librium, and the like? What about the pills that "everyone" takes when he cannot cope anymore, when adversity is too great? The anti-anxiety drugs reduce emotional reactions to the threats of adversity; that is why they are taken. Unfortunately, they also interfere with the body's ability to learn to tolerate stresses. That is why you never see a really tranquil person on tranquilizers!

Research into the use of these anti-anxiety pills has shown that there is an insidious danger in dependence on them. It has shown, first of all, that any adversity in our lives actually strengthens our character, allowing us to tolerate even greater adversity. An increased tolerance for stress develops simply as the result of the experience of stress and allows us to behave effectively under any subsequent stress. In other words, each time adversity faces us and we overcome it on our own we have grown stronger and better able to tolerate even greater stresses in the future. A body builder cannot have someone else lift heavy weights for him. He must do it himself if he is to grow stronger. Neither can we shun the responsibility of dealing with the stresses we have created in our lives. To do so would be to weaken our psychological resolve and make us captives to that weakness.

Anti-anxiety drugs reduce our reaction to what we perceive as stress, but at the same time they interfere with our ability to develop the appropriate response to it. The part of the brain that creates the emotional experience of "anxiety" in the first place is also the part that is charged with the function of decision-making to remove the anxiety! If one takes a pill to remove the emotion of anxiety, one will also blunt that part of the brain that is charged with making decisions for change. It may seem harmless to take an anti-anxiety drug to face the stresses of the day; but, in the long run, it is much wiser to develop behavior patterns to cope with these stresses because, when the effects of the pill wear off, the stress will still be there and will still have to be faced.

Coping with Stress

As with the answer to all questions, the answer to the question "How do I cope with stress?" is " . . . *seek first his kingdom. . . .* (Matt. 6:33) As long as we put God first in our lives, as long as we see ourselves as part of God and therefore part of good, as long as we consciously place ourselves in the flow of creation, we will have automatically lessened our stresses. Stress, worry, anxiety, and self-pity are examples of fear projected into the future. The more we center our thoughts on God and on good, the less fear we project, and the less stress we experience. Instead of looking to adversity for excuses, let us find comfort in the strength that it brings us.

Nutrients Help

A strong body is one that obeys. A weak body is one that commands. The weaker the body, the more attention it will demand; and the more attention our bodies demand, the fewer physical resources we will have available to adapt to stressful situations!

A sound body lives in silence. In order to develop a sound and silent body, attention must be paid to the raw materials we make available to the body for maintenance, repair, and renewal. In other words, in order for the body to be healthy it must have access to healthful foods.

Any discussion of maintaining, repairing, and renewing the body must begin with protein. Protein is the "mortar and bricks," the "wood and nails" which the life force uses to build and repair human tissue. It must have protein to do so. If we are interested in building a strong body structure, we should choose the finest proteins. (See chapter two, page 17.)

The main job of carbohydrates is to supply the body with fuel—with energy. In addition, carbohydrates assist the body in using fat properly and in supplying dietary fiber to ensure regular elimination.

Nature has provided us with some wonderful carbohydrates. They are fresh fruit (apples, bananas, melons, peaches, pears, etc.), fresh vegetables (squashes, green beans, salad greens, carrots, potatoes, etc.), and whole grains (wheat, rye, brown rice, corn, buckwheat, wild rice, oats, barley, etc., including baked products made with these grains). These are the only *constructive* carbohydrates. There are other carbohydrates but none that the body needs for optimum health.

The use of proper carbohydrates in the diet is of the utmost importance in overcoming a dependence on drugs. Probably the single biggest factor in drug abuse is the excessive ingestion of the destructive carbohydrates such as cola drinks, candy, cakes, highly-sugared desserts, and junk food of all kinds. Our bodies can only rebuild and renew with the raw materials we give them. If we feed them junk foods, what kind of health can we expect?

Watch your ingestion of carbohydrates. Use only the constructive ones, and you will feel the difference.

All machines need oil, and the miracle machine that we are is no exception. The best oils are unrefined vegetable oils. Particularly nutritious are safflower oil, sunflower oil, corn oil, and soy oil. These are best used raw.

Not so tasty, but particularly good for building a strong body, is wheat germ oil. This fine oil can improve physical performance. In athletes it increases endurance, lowers the pulse rate, improves the body's use of oxygen, and much more. Its taste makes it unsuitable for use in cooking, but it can be used in blender drinks, or it can be taken in capsule form. Try to get at least a teaspoonful each day. (Four 20 minim capsules equal one teaspoonful.)

Success with Supplements

Good nutrition begins with good foods. After ensuring that your food intake is nutritionally balanced, it is usually wise to supplement the diet with vitamins and minerals. This is particularly true in the case of those who have been abusing their bodies with drugs. Drugs, after all, are foreign to the body temple and force the body to eliminate, suspend, or speed up various natural functions. That is why they can be effective medicines. But to use them indiscriminately to perform tasks for which they were not designed is to inflict damage on the internal workings of the body and weaken its ability to respond vigorously to demands made on it.

A good place to start in your supplementation program is to take a strong multiple vitamin tablet and a multiple mineral tablet. These will ensure at least a minimum covering of all the nutritional "bases."

The two water-soluble vitamins, vitamins C and B complex, have very special application in cases of stress and/or drug abuse. The B complex vitamins are important because they are involved in helping the body to cope with stress and are essential to the health of the nerves.

Vitamin C, in addition to its important role in helping the body to cope with both physiological and psychological stresses, acts as a general detoxifying agent. In addition, it has a key role in the health of the adrenal glands—one of the major glands in our ability to respond to stresses.

Vitamin C is also important in fighting fatigue. It is essential for the absorption of iron and the use of B vitamins.

For anyone attempting to control drug abuse and to

cope with stress, a strong B complex vitamin once or twice a day and at least 3,000 milligrams of vitamin C might be a good idea.

The Liver Is the Hero

The liver is a key organ in overcoming drug abuse and in rebuilding the body. The liver is entrusted with the major responsibility of detoxifying the toxic effect of drugs. The liver does this heroically. So important is the liver, in fact, that the liver cells have been given the ability to regenerate themselves indefinitely! But, when the liver is abused, these cells begin to fill with fat and die. Certain substances, called lipotropics, are powerful fat-movers and have the ability to aid the liver cells. *In conjunction with a program of total nutrition,* lipotropic agents can help to rid the liver of this fat and renew it to its original state of health.

The primary lipotropic agents are choline, inositol (two B complex vitamins) and methionine (a constituent of top-grade protein foods). Often added are vitamin B12 and betaine. These lipotropics can be purchased in a single tablet at any health food store or drugstore.

The liver is one of the key organs, not only in a program designed to overcome drug dependence or stress, but for health in general. The health of the liver is primary to the health of the body. Anything that helps the liver helps the body. An axiom of ancient medicine is still true today: *similia similibus curantur* — like cures like.

It happens that one of the finest foods for the liver is liver! Liver can help to strengthen your own liver and other glands. It can help to overcome fatigue (and worry, anxiety, stress, and all other forms of fear-produced fatigue!); it also builds blood and is a fine protein-rich food.

Liver can provide you with a new spark of energy and

vitality while helping you to rebuild your body. Try eating it a few times a week. If you dislike liver, take desiccated liver tablets; but you may need to take ten to fifteen each day to take the place of the food.

Breakfast

All too many cases of drug abuse have been caused and exacerbated by poor nutritional habits. The reason for this is that of all the cells in the body, brain cells are the most dependent upon the minute-by-minute supply of glucose from the blood. What we eat, (or don't eat) especially at breakfast, directly affects the blood glucose level, and the blood glucose (or blood sugar) level directly affects the way we feel! When the blood glucose level gets too low (hypoglycemia) we can experience physical symptoms, such as headaches, weakness, cold sweats, fatigue, and inability to handle physical and/or emotional stress. Mental-emotional symptoms can include: depression, forgetfulness, confusion, nervousness, irritability, anxiety, difficulty in concentration, crying spells, and unidentifiable fears and apprehensions. In an effort to raise the blood glucose level, the tendency is to reach for something sweet—candy, a cola drink, cookies, or a stimulant, such as coffee. Alcohol is especially sought after because of its ability to raise the blood sugar very quickly. But the use of any of these gives only temporary results. Very shortly after ingesting any of these there is a quick decrease of blood sugar to an even lower level than before. This causes more severe symptoms. It is in such a state of physical, mental, and emotional discomfort that so many reach for a drug to make them feel good.

But good nutrition can make you feel good. (Those who suffer from the challenge of hypoglycemia—also called low blood sugar—would do well to read the chapter entitled "High Hopes for Hypoglycemia.") And the most important place to begin your good nutrition is with a nutritious breakfast. This is one of the real keys to health and to feeling vibrant and alive throughout the day. Breakfast does not have to be big to be good, but it should include *only* highly nutritious foods. Especially important are the top-grade proteins. Choose at least one of these, along with a good constructive carbohydrate. You will see the difference a good breakfast can make in the way you feel and act.

Exercise

Everyone knows that physical exercise has many benefits, but few realize that some of the most important benefits are in the area of mental health.

Exercise toughens us both physically and mentally. It improves our ability to withstand stress, and the stress that we may have already generated is released by exercise. The impulses generated in the spindles of the muscles during prolonged walking, for example, are essential to the optimum functioning of the central nervous system. The action of exercise can even absorb anxiety! (Why else would we pace the floor when we are nervous!)

Added to these benefits are the improvement of the cardio-vascular system and lungs, the increased circulation of the blood, the assistance to the lymphatic system, the aid to regular bowel movements, and the gentle massage to the inner muscles and organs of the body. These are just a few dividends that exercise can pay. There are many more.

Which exercise is best for you? Only you can decide. Walking, however, is good for virtually everyone. Brisk walking with arms swinging, and deep breathing, that is. The body was designed more for walking than for standing or sitting. Other good exercises are swimming, bicycling, aerobic dancing, and jogging. Find one that suits you and do it *regularly*.

Going Home

Any addiction, yours or that of someone you love, can be overcome. All dependency on outer things passes away when the soul is filled with the light of its own divinity. This is the knowing that satisfies the longing and lifts the spirits. The way becomes peace-filled and light. We begin to see life not "through a glass darkly" but with the clear vision of the eyes of God.

Perhaps you are reading this chapter not for yourself but with a loved one in mind. If so, it is important never to condemn, only to love.

Life is good. Life is beautiful. We can reach out to other souls and help lift them, too. We find meaning and goodness and joy wherever we look and in whatever we do. We sense a feeling of "being home." We are back in the Father's house, the source of all the good we could ever possibly want.

Jesus gave us a promise which is too wonderful not to accept. He said: " . . . *seek first his kingdom and his righteousness, and all these things shall be yours as well."* (Matt. 6:33) Accept that promise now. Start working on it. Get to know what it feels like to be a child of God.

Within you is the divine power to lift you higher than any drugs. Within you is an eternal wellspring of living waters which, once drunk, will satisfy all thirst for "something more." Within you is a mighty life force which is working for your wholeness.

The Father is holding "open house" for you right this moment. A feast is waiting. It is a perpetual invitation. Go in. Take the step across the threshold. *This* is what you were hungering for: It was God all along! Welcome home, dear one. Welcome home.

The Story on Skin

When Moses came down from Mount Sinai . . . the skin of his face shone . . . . (Exod. 34:29)

Have you ever noticed that whenever you are happy and filled with a sense of peace and total trust in God your face shines? Do you know people who are so centered in their awareness of the presence of God that their skin has taken on a radiant look? This is quite logical when you realize that the skin always reflects what is going on inside, mentally and physically. Our skin is the only part of us that we can show to the world.

What an astounding organ (yes, it is the largest organ of the body) the skin is! It exists not only to give the body its outer appearance, but it is also a vibrant gatherer of endless data about our environment. The skin flexes and folds its way across the body structure and is studded with a half million tiny transmitters all poised and waiting to rush important news to the brain.

This covering, which protects us from the outside world, serves many purposes. It warns us of dangers, registers heat and cold, carries off impurities, and is our first line of defense when it comes to keeping our bodies healthy.

Elastic Armor

The skin is like a flexible suit of armor which, as long as it is unbroken, guards against foreign invaders. No germs, bacteria, or infections can enter the unbroken skin, and this one small provision of the Creator is one of the most remarkable strengths we possess. The skin is so strong that it takes a very long period of time submerged in water before even a tiny amount of that water will be absorbed by the body through the skin.

In general, it is very difficult for anything to penetrate these elastic walls of the body temple. In fact, aside from taking up sunlight, the skin always works from within out!

More Than Skin Deep

To understand more fully the role and the significance of the skin, let us examine some metaphysical ideas that have been ascribed to the skin and its problems.

The skin symbolizes divine protection. It is the protective covering of the deeper tissues of the body. It is quickly responsive to outer conditions and ever sensitive to the life within. Your reaction to the atmosphere of the world about you as well as to the radiation of light from the inner Christ realm has much to do with the condition of your skin. So says Clara Palmer in *You Can Be Healed.*

Being such a responsive barometer of our inner and outer world, we can look to the skin for first signs when something is awry. Problems with the skin can denote a sense of threat, a sense of insecurity, an impatience with things as they are.

A rash may be a way of getting attention; acne can stem from a dislike and nonacceptance of one's self; eczema is often traced to an overly-sensitive nature; psoriasis may have its roots in a sense of emotional insecurity. Naturally, these metaphysical interpretations are general and do not apply in every case. However, if one is suffering from a skin problem, it would seem wise to at least consider these interpretations—to at least "try them on for size."

Spiritualize the Skin

The skin holds together the body temple. It is fitting, therefore, that we help it to be as beautiful and wholesome as it can possibly be. The skin is our individual physical identity. No two people look *exactly* alike. Each of us has his own unique set of fingerprints. God fashioned each of us in a very special way. *"Thou didst clothe me with skin and flesh. . . . "* (Job 10:11)

If you find yourself with skin that is less desirable than you would like it to be, there is much you can do about it! With God as your partner you can refashion your skin into the radiant mantle it was designed to be.

The first step in correcting the condition is meditation. During regularly scheduled daily sessions of contacting your inner Source of life and health, picture the old condition as completely gone. Image your skin as radiantly, glowingly perfect. See yourself covered by smooth, resilient, comfortable skin. See yourself free of all imperfections. Make the image of perfect skin as real as you can, and hold that image for as long as you can.

Using this technique it is even possible to get rid of some scars, birthmarks, discolorations, and other imperfections through lifting our minds to a higher level of consciousness. The fact is that new skin cells are constantly being born, replacing old ones. We do not have to let our negative thoughts continue to mold these new cells into the old conditions. Think positive! Think new! Think radiance! Think life, and think love! Think God!

Through persistent imaging in your meditative times, you can bring these newborn skin cells into an environment

289

of wholeness and beauty. Keep in mind that your rewards will match your efforts, and so regular application of high-level thoughts and imaging is necessary.

If you are willing to make the effort, you can improve your skin. Meditation and prayer are the basis of your effort. We always begin with God first and work at aligning ourselves with the Creator's healing, perfecting power.

Foods to Save Face

Any talk of foods to improve the skin must begin with protein. Protein plays a crucial role in the makeup of the two main layers of skin: the outer epidermis and the thicker, underlying dermis.

The epidermis contains a tough outer fabric of dead cells. Much like the shingles on the roofs of our homes, they are the first to take the abuse of sun, rain, cold, and heat. They are constantly flaking and being rubbed away. However, the epidermis also contains living cells. These cells are constantly migrating outward, filling en route with keratin, an indigestable, insoluble, and very durable protein (also found in hair and nails). In this way the outer "shingles" are always being replaced. It is almost like having a perpetually new roof put on from the inside out!

The dermis is a very busy area. It contains a complex collection of sweat glands, blood and lymphatic vessels, nerve endings, and hair follicles. But it is the network of protein fibers in the dermis around which all these are built which gives the skin its strength and elasticity.

The protein ingested should be of the highest quality. Strict vegetarians who eat nothing from animal or dairy products must be careful to combine their other incomplete foods properly to create top quality protein foods. For example, legumes, if eaten exclusively, cannot build new high-quality tissue. Nor can grains, if eaten alone. However, when the two are combined (such as beans and rice) they create a complete protein capable of consistently building strong tissue, including skin tissue.

The body also needs carbohydrates if it is to be healthy. Carbohydrates are its source of energy. In seeking healthy skin it is important to eat constructive carbohydrates. In fact, *the ingestion of the destructive carbohydrates has more to do with skin problems than perhaps any other single physical cause.* Destructive carbohydrates cause internal pollution which the body throws off via the skin and other organs of elimination.

The constructive carbohydrates are fresh fruit, fresh vegetables, and whole grains. If sweeteners are desired, it is best to use very small amounts of honey or blackstrap molasses. If your skin problem is acne, no sweeteners should be used. Those with acne should also keep away from high-sugared fruit such as citrus, which is about ten percent natural sugar. Grapes may also be too sweet. Also avoid coffee, alcohol, chocolate, and cocoa as well as all candy, cola drinks, soft drinks, diet drinks, and baked products made with sugar.

Dried fruits and fruit juices, because they are so very concentrated in the natural fruit sugars, should also be avoided. (Special note: Artificial sweeteners can only build artificial health.)

Fats are important for the skin but not necessarily the saturated fats found in animal products. The skin and the rest of the body need the highly unsaturated fats found in vegetable oils such as safflower oil, sunflower oil, corn oil, and soy oil. When using these oils do not use them for frying. Use them raw on salads, baked potatoes, vegetables, and in blender drinks; use them wherever you can. Buy them without preservatives. Often the only place you can

291

purchase such unchemicalized oils is at a health food store. Be sure to refrigerate after opening. Try to get one or two teaspoonsful of one of these wonderful oils each day.

Also important but not so tasty are cod liver oil, high in vitamins A and D, and wheat germ oil. Both are very nutritious, and both come in capsule form.

Good nutrition begins with good food, and we should make every effort to get the finest foods into our diet every day. However, there are times when we have allowed our bodies to get to a point when food alone, no matter how healthful, is not enough. This is often true in problems with the skin.

Therefore, it is generally a good idea to supplement the diet with extra vitamins and minerals. Remember, vitamins and minerals are natural constituents of God's foods, and the body anxiously accepts them and joyously uses them to build more vibrant health.

A good program of supplementation begins with a well-rounded, complete vitamin-mineral supplement, one with generous amounts of vitamin A and the B complex, and with at least a small amount of minerals.

Vitamin A is essential for the integrity of the epithelial system, of which the skin is the largest part. So important is vitamin A for the skin that Dr. Hans van Eys, head of the Department of Pediatrics at MD Anderson Hospital and Tumor Institute, wrote in the "Journal of Applied Nutrition": *If anyone gets enough vitamin A, it would be almost impossible to have cancer of the skin and mouth.* Now please read this carefully! Dr. van Eys is not saying that vitamin A cures skin cancer. He is merely stating that if the tissues in the skin and mouth have sufficient vitamin A it is unlikely that cancer will develop.

We should be sure that this important vitamin is generously supplied in the diet and/or as a supplement. Good food sources are liver, eggs, green leafy vegetables, carrots, yellow squashes, sweet potatoes, prunes, apricots, avocados, and yellow peaches. If supplementation is desired, it is often best to use the dry or aqueous form of vitamin A to ensure adequate digestion. The body has the ability to store vitamin A, so do not overdo your intake of supplemental vitamin A. Do not think that because a little will do you good, a lot will do better. It won't! Concentrate on getting your vitamin A in God's fine foods, and if you feel you should supplement, use between 25,000 and 50,000 I.U.'s each day.

A good B complex vitamin may also be needed since forms of dermatitis are symptoms of many B complex deficiencies. In cases of acne, additional amounts of B6 may also be needed. (But be sure to take the entire B complex too!) The B vitamins work best as a family, so check to see that yours is complete, with all eleven of the B's present in the tablet.

Because of the function of vitamin E as an antioxidant and its ability to control the destruction of "free radicals" in the body which cause wrinkles and aging skin, extra vitamin E is also an important supplement for healthy skin. In addition, vitamin E helps to protect vitamin A.

Vitamin C is also an antioxidant and is responsible for making the "cement" which holds the skin together. Many knowledgeable scientists feel that 3,000 milligrams per day is a minimum amount needed for vibrant health.

Important, too, are minerals, especially calcium. It may be wise to take a supplemental multiple-mineral tablet which contains about 1,000 milligrams of calcium plus all the other major and trace elements.

Rounding out your supplements with a tablespoonful of lecithin granules (3 or more tablespoonsful per day for cases of psoriasis) would put you well on your way to vi-

293

brant skin and vibrant health.

Moving Toward Success

The finest nutrition in the world will do little to improve the skin if the nutrients are unable to reach it! And nothing improves the delivery of nutrients to all parts of the body better than exercise. In fact, exercise, done regularly, has as much to do with vibrant health as any other single factor.

For healthier skin choose an exercise that can be done out of doors in the fresh air. Walking is always a good choice. One hour of brisk walking daily (or at least four times per week) will make a difference in your health. But also excellent are exercises such as swimming, bicycling, jogging, rope jumping, yoga, and many others. Any movement brings improvement, but to make it most meaningful, do it regularly.

Sun and Skin

The sun is the skin's best friend and its worst enemy! Sunlight reacts with a substance on the skin to form vitamin D, which is essential for calcium absorption, which in turn is essential for healthy skin. In a sense, the skin looks to the sun for food! Those with acne can derive great benefit from moderate exposure to sunlight, as can many with psoriasis. But this warm, beautiful sunlight must be used in great moderation. Long periods of exposure to the sun do more to damage the skin than any other factor. Nothing ages skin faster than too much sunlight. That deep tan might look good temporarily, but since the deleterious effects of the sun are cumulative over our entire lifetime, it is not worth the price your skin must pay.

It is the ultraviolet rays of the sun that do the most

damage to the skin. In fact, these rays are responsible for the vast majority of skin cancers. And one does not have to be exposed directly to the sun to be exposed to the sun's ultraviolet rays. You can be sitting on the beach under an umbrella, feeling cool, while your skin is actually roasting! The sun's infrared rays, which you would feel as heat, are being shielded by the umbrella. However, the ultraviolet rays, which cause sunburn and other damage, including skin cancer, come at you from all directions. They come at you from the sky and from sand or water reflection. In fact, the amount of ultraviolet radiation from the sky is greater than that coming directly from the sun!

Try to keep out of the sun between 10 a.m. and 2 p.m. If you are on vacation or working in the sun, use a good sunscreen. Sunscreens are rated from one to fifteen. A product labeled one gives the least protection. One labeled fifteen offers the greatest protection; in fact, it acts as a virtual sun block, filtering out almost all harmful ultraviolet rays.

Take care of your skin while in the sun. Wear a broad-brimmed hat and use a sunscreening agent. Many foundation makeups contain them. It is wise to use them, especially if you are fair-skinned.

Treat the sun with respect. Remember, the sun is food for the skin. Don't overeat!

A New Face

You know now that it is not necessary to have poor skin. Isn't it good to feel that you can do something about the condition? Through regular meditation, through imaging, through proper nutrition, and through a program of physical exercise, you will be able to present a new face to the world and a new covering for your holy body temple.

Having good skin is actually one way of praising God, because it provides your indwelling divinity with an exterior befitting the Almighty.

As your skin is regenerated into its intended beautiful state, you will feel good about yourself and your role in the universal scheme of things.

God devised your marvelous skin to serve you well. Let your skin reflect the vitality and radiance of your inner spirit. Bless your skin. God adorned you with it so that you can express uniquely in your world. *"Thus says the Lord God . . . I . . . will cause flesh to come upon you, and cover you with skin, and put breath in you, and you shall live; and you shall know that I am the Lord."* (Ezek. 37:5, 6)

The Cancer Challenge

What a marvel of creation is the human body! Beginning as a solitary cell nestled deep within a mother's womb, it is majestically transformed, in a period of just nine months, from its microscopic solitude into a living, breathing, moving, thinking expression of its Creator. By the time it reaches full maturity a few decades later, the one cell will have grown into 100 trillion cells, each working unselfishly for the good of the entire body. Some cells will agree to form a heart and will begin pulsating 100,000 times each day, pumping 7,000 quarts of life-giving blood to all the other cells. Others will have differentiated into kidneys complete with two million filtering units, filter sheets, strainers, and reabsorption mechanisms. These diminutive high-pressure filters will be capable of filtering out 200 quarts per day of the waste products of all the cells' metabolism. Other cells will form the blood vessels, arteries, and capillaries—a system of pipes and conduits stretching out over 60,000 miles in length! Added to these are the specialized muscle cells, bone cells, the unique cells of the organs and tissues and, finally, the climax of evolution, the human brain—sixteen billion cells which are the central switchboard in the most complex, complete, and awe-inspiring communication network in creation. It is impossible to imagine the Mind capable of designing all of this!

As long as each of the 100 trillion cells of the human body follows its divine design, the body sings in harmony to the melody of life. But what happens when, for one reason or another, the cells lose their body wisdom and begin to act not in accordance with the good of the body but to the body's detriment? We call such action on the part of the cells "sickness" or "disease."

One such "dis-ease" is cancer. Cancer cells are cells that have lost their body wisdom; they have lost the ability to perform all the functions of the cells except one—the ability to reproduce. It is because of this singularity of purpose, this obsession with reproducing, that these cells need to be purged from the body.

Let us assert at the outset that only you can determine which path to follow in seeking healing. There is no suggestion whatsoever on the part of the authors or UNITY Books that you should avoid medical treatment. By all means, see a physician if you suspect cancer. *All* healing is of God. The hands of the physician are working just as much on behalf of your inner life force as is your most spiritual affirmation. We offer this information merely as a tool. It is entirely up to you as to how much of it (if any) you wish to work with. You must make your effort where your faith is, because it is ultimately your belief that brings about the effect. If your belief is in your physician, well and good. It does not mean, however, that you must exclude the ideas presented here. Be open to your good, no matter from which direction it comes.

It is unfortunate that because of the stories we hear, or because we may have lost loved ones from it, cancer is thought to be a capriciously inflicted foreign invader capable of unstoppable destruction and death. But from a strictly scientific viewpoint (not to mention the metaphysical implications!) this is far from true. Cancer cells are not the strong, unyielding juggernauts of doom that their reputation suggests. They are, in fact, very weak, primitive, disorganized, and confused cells very much out of place in our well-organized body temples. This point is important to remember because this disorder, this anarchy of the cancer cells, is their very vulnerability. Those who are faced with this challenge can take advantage of the internal chaos among cancer cells. But they can do so only when they have a singularity of purpose, only when they have a firm goal in mind, only when their desire to overcome cancer is stronger, more focused, and more determined than the cancer cell's desire to reproduce.

Scientifically Speaking

Let's take a minute to examine cancer from a physiological point of view. There are many secondary causes of cancer, more are being discovered yearly; but there is only one prime biochemical cause, and that is the replacement of oxygen in the respiratory chemistry of normal cells by the fermentation of sugar. What does this mean?

All cells need energy. Normal cells utilize oxygen from the air we breathe to convert blood sugar into energy. Oxygen is the basis of life on this planet. However, there is another way to make energy, and this process does not need oxygen. It is a more primitive, anaerobic (without oxygen) process called fermentation. It is the process used by malignant cells.

Cancer cells are not truly foreign bodies. They are normal cells that have changed their utilization of energy by conversion to a more primitive state used in earlier stages of evolution. In this lower state, all powers have been lost to the cell except the most basic and primitive power—that of reproduction. Of course, in their unrestrained frenzy of reproduction, the cancer cells crowd out and disrupt the healthy cells and work at cross purposes to the health of the body.

299

Cancer Is the Effect

Like any other dis-ease, cancer is an effect. We must ask ourselves "what is the cause?" No matter how basic and primary any *physical* cause is, we know that it is always secondary to the real cause, which is always *metaphysical*—beyond the physical. Before a malignancy shows up on X-ray film, it must first have been a malignancy in our minds—in our thinking.

And what are some of the "mental malignancies" that are capable of prompting such an unwanted response in our bodies? Among the most insidious offenders are such feelings as hatred, unforgiveness, resentment, jealousy, envy, and malevolent feelings of any sort. Can such seeds, when planted in the fertile soil of our consciousness, ripen into anything but the bitter fruit of disease and disharmony in our bodies? What of the hatred or resentment we feel toward another? Doesn't it, after a short time, have a life of its own? Doesn't it reproduce? Doesn't it fester and grow, rejecting all restraints, crowding out other thoughts of harmony and love?

Are we caught up in a chaos of unforgiveness? Have we reverted to a lower and more primitive state in our relationships with others? Do we follow the strict, unforgiving admonitions used in an earlier state of evolution or consciousness which told us *an eye for an eye?* (Matt. 5:38) Or do we follow the New Testament or new consciousness precepts that tell us to *turn the other cheek,* (Matt. 5:39) to forgive *seventy times seven,* (Matt. 18:22) and that *the greatest of these is love?* (I Cor. 13:13)

There can be no permanent healing of the body without a corresponding healing of our thoughts and emotions. Just as malignant cells are normal cells that have lost their ability to utilize oxygen, a basic element of life on this

300

planet, so malignant thoughts mirror a consciousness that has lost its ability to utilize love—the basic element of life in creation! Love is the oxygen of spiritual growth, and spiritual growth is the basis of physical health. Unless love, given generously and unconditionally, is in our lives, we will forever wallow in the primitive darkness of unhappiness in our lives and affairs. Consciousness cannot be changed by radiation, surgery, or chemicals. These can remove cancer from the body but not from the mind. And as long as the consciousness harbors such disharmonious seeds, the potential for disease exists.

After the man at the pool of Bethzatha changed his consciousness and was healed, Jesus admonished him: " . . . *See, you are well! Sin no more, that nothing worse befall you.*" (John 5:14) In other words, "Be aware of the fact that your consciousness is changed and that this changed consciousness has made you well. Now keep it changed so that you think only thoughts of God and of good. If you go back to your old way of thinking, the same sickness, or worse, will come into your life."

Disharmonious thoughts affect the body in very definite ways. The stresses caused by hatred, unforgiveness, resentment, and by lack of love in general are measurable and quantifiable. Such feelings carry with them outrageous physical and emotional price tags. When these feelings are prolonged, stress accumulates in the body. With no outlet, the body has no chance to regenerate. The constant stress caused by jealousy, anger, rage, hatred, and unforgiveness or simply by lack of love is like racing your car's engine with one foot on the gas pedal and the other on the brake. Sooner or later something has to give.

The Price of Stress

Emotional stress is no different than physical stress as far as body reactions are concerned. Both, in fact, lower the body's resistance to disease. There is a very clear link between stress and illness, between emotional states and the health of the body.

In his inspiring and informative book "Getting Well Again," Dr. Carl Simonton states: *It is our central premise that an illness is not purely a physical problem but rather a problem of the whole person, that it includes not only body but mind and emotions. We believe that emotional and mental states play a significant role both in susceptibility to disease, including cancer, and in recovery from all disease. We believe that cancer is often an indication of problems elsewhere in an individual's life, problems aggravated or compounded by a series of stresses six to eighteen months prior to the onset of cancer."*

Dr. Simonton's premise becomes more obvious when one realizes that chronic stress produces measurable hormonal imbalances and suppresses the body's immune system. The immune system is one of our first lines of defense and the mortal enemy of cancer cells. Normal cells are always, in small numbers, turning malignant. One of the prime tasks of the immune system is to search them out, identify them, and destroy them. When the immune system is unencumbered by chronic negative thoughts, this is done routinely, almost daily. When negative thoughts predominate, however, the immune system is unable to perform at its optimum level.

So the real first line of defense in the body is our emotional health! If we are emotionally healthy, we will be physically healthy. Body and mind are not two separate entities; they are one. And when our thoughts are of God and good, our actions will follow and our bodies and affairs will mirror this good.

Attitude

Attitude is all-important. You must actively participate in your health as much as you do in your sickness. If you are faced with a cancer challenge, what should you do? The first thing to do is to ask yourself the question, "Do I want to be healed?" It may sound like a foolish question, but it is not. Subconsciously or consciously we all have chosen the things that are in our lives. Everything touching our lives is there for a reason. When we discover the reason and learn whatever lesson we need from it, we can release it, and it will disappear. In asking yourself, "Do I want to be healed" you are really asking, "Have I discovered yet why this challenge is in my life and, having discovered it, am I ready to change so that it can leave?"

What aspects of you need this challenge? Do you feel you deserve to be healed? Do you feel worthy? How would you act if you were healed tomorrow? How would you feel next year or five years from now? Is your life meaningful without such a challenge? As Dr. Arnold Hutschnecker says in his classic book "The Will to Live" (not available from Unity): *We may have a reason to live without the wish to live, and when reason and emotion are locked in battle . . . emotion eventually wins.*

Ask yourself these questions in quiet meditation. The answers must be honest. They must flow from deep within, from that part of you that knows your most secret motives. The penalty for lying to the world is often severe, but the penalty for lying to yourself is always disastrous!

Evaluation

Next, you must ask, "What do I have to change in order to rid myself of this challenge?" The easiest way to discern this is to identify those aspects of your life with which you are most dissatisfied—those that are the most stressful to you. These will be the areas that need change.

Is there a personal relationship that needs work? Is there less than unconditional love flowing from you to those in your life? Don't worry about others hating you; that is their problem, not yours. So long as you love them generously, graciously, and unconditionally, so long as you *"sin no more,"* you have done your perfect work and you will be rewarded.

It is important to realize that sickness is not the opposite of health—sickness is *congested* health. And there is only one way to treat congestion, and that is with circulation. Love, circulated freely, given unconditionally, breaks up this congestion and allows you to claim your wholeness. Love is the great emancipator. Love is your miracle drug.

Imagination

It is important to remember that you were created perfect. Often, when faced with a serious challenge, this is easy to forget. In God's realm there exist no sickness, disease, or death. Within you flows a life force which was conceived in God's realm and which is part of every cell, tissue, muscle, bone, nerve, organ, and system in your body. Because it was conceived and nurtured in God's realm, it too knows nothing of sickness or death. It knows only life and seeks only life. As Charles Fillmore wrote: *The vital energy of eternal life exists in every cell of our body.* When you feel that this life force, this *vital energy of eternal life,* is no longer flowing freely, if you feel it has been inhibited by your thoughts and actions, you can use one of the most dynamic of your powers to reawaken this life force and begin its flowing again. That power, of course, is the wonderful power of imagination.

A period of *regular, daily* imaging is one of the most important and fulfilling pursuits you can follow. Spend time (at least two sessions each day) imaging your cells following their divine plan of mutual help. *See* the life force flowing through all the cells, strengthening the normal ones, and washing away the weak and confused ones. *See* the body's immune system working with this life force, performing the task that the Creator entrusted it with—that of removing any destructive cells from the body just as you will be removing any destructive thoughts from your mind. (You can actually increase the number of lymphocytes—the white blood cell "soldiers" that destroy foreign and harmful cells—by the use of imagination, as tests at Penn State have proven.) Use your imagination in any way you feel comfortable. It is a powerful tool that can be used to build a strong consciousness of health.

Denial

A denial is a tool that can be used to remove from your consciousness any beliefs not consistent with Truth. This is not to say you can use a denial to manipulate outer reality. A denial such as *pain and sickness are not real and cannot affect me* does not imply that you have never felt pain and sickness. What it really means is that these conditions do not have reality, power, or dominion of their own. Therefore, they cannot have reality, power, or dominion in your life unless you allow them these traits.

That unnatural tissue mass appearing on the X ray of a

man's lung cannot be denied; it clearly shows on the film! He cannot really believe a denial such as *I no longer have cancer.* But he can deny the *inevitability* of the tissue mass to remain in the body. He can deny the *power* of this mass to affect him any longer. He can deny any *dominion* that this mass can have over his life. He can say and truly believe: *I no longer need this problem.* He can say and truly believe: *These cells have no power over me.* When he denies this disease any dominion or power over him, he cuts out its root system and robs it of all nourishment. Without the nourishment of his negative thoughts the tissue mass will waste away until it completely disappears. Therefore, rather than being in his lungs, the "reality" of the disease would have been in his mind!

When you repeat a denial, you are not denying the appearance of a situation, *you are denying the reality of those appearances,* and denying them any power over you.

Make up a special denial that suits you. Often, in the case of a stubborn situation, there can be no better denial than a powerful, loud, and insistent "no!" each time a negative thought or emotion tries to intrude. Whatever denial you decide upon, make it short, specific, and meaningful to you. Repeat it as often as you can throughout the day and mean what you say.

Affirmations

Denials must be followed by affirmations if you are to be successful in changing your consciousness. Affirmative statements *based on Truth* help you to claim the wholeness that is yours by divine right. Statements such as *God is healing me now,* or *I allow the life force to express as a perfect body,* or any other statement based on Truth and repeated throughout the day will imbed the idea in your consciousness. As with denials, make your affirmation short and specific—one that has a good "ring" to it deep within your soul.

You can only become what you believe yourself to be. Denials and affirmations help you to see more clearly what you really are.

True Prayer

In praying for a healing, what is your *true* prayer? Are you begging God to remove that tumor from your lungs while you continue to smoke? Are you beseeching God for help with your liver but still drinking alcohol? You may be praying for deliverance from your challenge, but if your daily actions are inconsistent with health, you should realize that your *true* prayers—your actions—are not for health at all!

Are your deeds consistent with your desires? Evaluate them. Your words and thoughts are your desires, but your deeds are your *true* prayers. A desire without a deed is a dead end. Be sure you attach the appropriate deeds to your most fervent desires. In most cases this will mean a complete change in life-style in order to attune yourself with the flow of the universe.

Experiment after experiment shows a correlation between diet and cancer. A good place to begin your deeds is in the area of nutrition. Remember, you are a population of 100 trillion cells. Each cell is a chemical factory that needs raw material in order to function properly. Nutrition presents the cells with this raw material. Good nutrition, of course, begins with good food, and the good foods are the primary proteins, the constructive carbohydrates, and the essential fatty acids God has provided.

Protein

Renewing and rebuilding the body requires protein. This is the "bricks and mortar" of our tissues. Although many foods contain protein, there are only certain foods balanced enough to be called complete proteins. (See chapter two, page 17, for listing.)

Carbohydrates

Supplying the body with energy is the main (but not the only) function of constructive carbohydrates. Another important role that carbohydrates fulfill is that of presenting the body with sufficient dietary fiber, so important for regular elimination and for preventing many problems in the colon.

The word "constructive" is very important when dealing with carbohydrates because the non-constructive carbohydrates have more to do with encouraging and exacerbating disease, including cancer, than any other single physical cause. Many researchers point the finger at sugar, white flour, soft drinks, diet drinks, high calorie snacks, and overly refined "junk" foods of all kinds. Experiments show a high correlation between the ingestion of these "destructive" carbohydrates and cancer.

On the other hand, tests which have supplied all known nutrients, including the constructive carbohydrates, have resulted in major successes in preventing and curing cancer.

And what are the constructive carbohydrates? They are fresh fruits, fresh vegetables, and whole grains. These are the carbohydrates with which the life force works most efficiently. These are the carbohydrates that contain the microscopic elements needed for each cell in our bodies.

Within this seemingly small group there is a plethora of wonderful choices. Apples, pears, peaches, melons, bananas, and many others are wholesome, delicious fruits. Among the fine vegetables are salad greens, squashes, potatoes, peas, green beans, and many more. The wonderful whole grains include wheat, rye, millet, brown rice, buckwheat, corn, oats, and barley. (These may be eaten in the form of whole-grain baked goods, cereals, or simply cooked alone.)

If sweeteners are needed, small amounts of honey, blackstrap molasses, and pure maple syrup may be used. (Artificial sweeteners cannot be used by the life force and should not be eaten. At best they can bring only artificial health!)

Essential Fatty Acids

Essential fatty acids are also needed by the body. The finest source of these is in refined vegetable oils such as safflower, sunflower, corn, soy, and sesame. These tasty oils can be used on salads, baked potatoes, and other foods. It is best to use them raw and unheated.

Not so tasty, but wonderfully nutritious, are cod liver oil and wheat germ oil. Both of these oils are highly unsaturated and have very special significance in the health of the body. (Although animal fats contain fatty acids, they are of a saturated, non-essential type that the body does not need and, in fact, excessive amounts of them are very harmful. While facing a cancer challenge it may be wise to discontinue the use of muscle meats, although organ meats are acceptable.)

Nuts and seeds (raw and unsalted) are excellent sources of good fatty acids and other nutrients and make wonderful snacks.

Good nutrition strengthens the body so that it is able to withstand aggravation by carcinogens. Good nutrition also strengthens the immune system—cancer's mortal enemy. And keep in mind that good nutrition begins with God's good foods.

However, when there is a serious challenge to the body, as in the case of cancer, it is always appropriate to augment good nutrition with suitable amounts of nutritional supplements. Writing in the "Journal of Applied Nutrition," Dr. John Myers states: *Supplementation of the diet throughout life with vitamins and minerals to support the oxygen respiration cycle of the cell is recommended as a preventive measure against cancer . . . good health, free of cancer . . . is produced by diet containing adequate and balanced vitamins and minerals. . . .*

Such a program of supplementation begins with a strong, complete multiple vitamin tablet (or tablets) containing all the vitamins.

Add to this multiple vitamin A, since it has a role in the proper functioning of the immune system and is especially important in protecting against cancers of the mouth, skin, and epithelial tissues. (Since vitamin A is stored in the body it is not wise to take high amounts for long periods of time.)

Since vitamin E works right along with vitamin A, and since it actually reduces the oxygen utilization by the tissues, it too is an important supplement.

The B complex vitamins are needed in much greater amounts than normal, especially in light of the fact that they act as a powerful activator of the immune system. (Deficiencies of the B complex actually suppress the immune system.) The B vitamins are also absolutely essential for oxygen transfer in the cells. The B complex is not complete without all eleven of its members. Make certain that the one you select contains them all.

Vitamin C has been shown effective in many experiments in both prevention of cancer and in the treatment of established cancers. It is one of the most important of the supplements. It, too, potentiates the immune system, strengthening it and preparing it to rid the body of "outlaw" cells. Vitamin C also has the ability to help detoxify many carcinogens. Not only that, vitamin C has been found to lessen X ray sickness (as have the B complex vitamins). Dr. Ewan Cameron and Nobel prizewinner Dr. Linus Pauling state: *It is our conclusion that this simple and safe treatment, the ingestion of large amounts of vitamin C, is of definite value in the treatment of patients with advanced cancer . . . we believe that vitamin C has even greater value for the treatment of patients with the disease in earlier stages and also for the prevention of cancer.* Drs. Cameron and Pauling's experiments were carried out using 10,000 milligrams (10 grams) of vitamin C per day—an amount they feel is minimum.

A multiple mineral tablet containing all the major and trace minerals would round out the supplement program.

Remember, *complete* nutrition is what you are seeking. Such good nutrition keeps the 100 trillion cells healthy and functioning to provide energy and to build and repair tissue and, in regard to carcinogens, to detoxify those that cannot be eliminated.

Your eating of good food should reflect your desire to build the finest body temple. It should not be done out of fear of what will happen if you don't. When your concern is to build the finest temple, your actions will mirror your desire, and you will automatically choose only wholesome foods.

Exercise

It is clear that prolonged stress inhibits the life force and harms the body. It does so both by sustaining tension and expending unnecessary energy. In such a weakened state, the body is much more susceptible to disease. When animals are chronically stressed and not permitted a physical outlet, there is a deterioration of their bodies. However, when stressed and allowed to exercise, the damage is minimal. Physical exercise can calm and soothe the nerves. It can, and will, alleviate stress. Exercise acts as an emergency valve which allows you to "let off steam."

One of the finest exercises for accomplishing this is walking. Regular, vigorous walking is nature's antidote for stress. It is believed that the impulses generated in the spindles of the muscles during prolonged walking are essential to the optimum functioning of our central nervous system. Walking, of course, is not the only good exercise. Such endeavors as cycling, swimming, yoga, tennis, golf, jogging, and countless others can also be effective. The point is, do something!

Exercise done *regularly and joyfully* brings many other benefits as well as alleviating stress. First of all, exercise will bring more oxygen to the waiting cells. With sufficient oxygen, the cells will have less need to revert to the more primitive methods of energy production.

Secondly, and more subtly, it makes you take more control of your life. When you are making a regular effort on your own behalf, this will indicate to you that you have decided to take control of your own destiny. The discipline of an exercise regime will help convince you and the life force that you really mean business.

Thirdly, regular exercise teaches you to "listen" to your body, to be responsive to what it is telling you about your

312

life—inside, outside, and all around you.

And, lastly, exercise will motivate you. The steady improvement you will observe will be a constant reminder of how much better you can feel as long as you continue making an effort on your own behalf.

Choose an exercise that suits you best and do it cheerfully, enthusiastically, and regularly.

Meditation

No matter how hectic your life has become, *time must be set aside each day for quiet meditation.* The benefits from this daily experience cannot be overestimated. Remembering that the life force within you knows nothing about disease, decay, or death—that it knows only life and seeks only life—reserve at least twenty to thirty minutes each day to make contact with that life force and learn how you can best work with it. It is usually more effective to set apart the same time each day so that there will develop an air of expectancy each time you prepare to meditate.

And do not forget to spend additional time on your mental imagery process. Use your imagination to direct healing forces throughout your entire body. Your imagination is one of the most powerful and important tools you can bring into your self-healing.

All those who have conquered cancer or any other disease have one thing in common—*a positive expectancy*—the belief that they can exert a positive influence over their health challenge. Deep within our souls we know that it is faith, not time, which determines when a cure will be effected, and faith can be increased in some very subtle ways.

First of all, act as if you want to be well. Act as if you want this cancer challenge out of your life. Make your every

313

deed reflect this desire.

Surround yourself with happy things, with flowers, funny cartoons, inspirational music, and happy people. Watch only uplifting programs on television, and read only positive books. Let your every action be toward improving yourself.

Charles Fillmore once wrote: *. . . cancers, tumors, and the many other ills of the flesh are evidences that nature has been outraged and is protesting and striving to free itself from its unhappy condition.*

Every cell of the body is enveloped in soul or thought, and its initial impulse is to conform to the divine-natural law.

Don't inhibit this impulse of your cells by talking about "my" cancer or anyone else's cancer. It is not "your" cancer unless and until you embrace it as yours. Too often, when one is told that he has cancer, it becomes his defining characteristic. One is no longer a husband or a wife or a father or a mother or a lawyer or an accountant or a secretary. One is a "cancer victim!" That and that alone becomes his overriding identity. "My" cancer becomes one's whole life.

Mr. Fillmore wrote in *Jesus Christ Heals: God created man in His image, in the image of perfect health.* To think otherwise is to give cancer too much dominion. Such an attitude will not only pervert your fully human identity but, worse than that, it will hide from you your divine identity. You are an individualized expression of God, and that is your only *real* characteristic. Dwelling on this Truth will activate and strengthen the life force within you and allow you to express the wholeness that is yours by divine inheritance.

Charles Fillmore often spoke of the physical cells in the body as being either light-filled or dark. *In good health there is a preponderance of the light cells; in ill health the dark cells predominate. . . . Man can light up the body cells by affirming life and intelligence for them. . . .* It is our respon-

314

sibility to regenerate these dark cells: *. . . until finally every cell becomes so related to its neighbor that each reflects the other, as diamond reflects diamond, and the redeemed body literally shines.*

Cancer, like any challenge, is not based on Truth. It is only what we make it. When we step back into the flow of life, learning and obeying *all* the divine laws (spiritual, mental, and physical) which our Creator designed for us, we find ourselves harmonized. The darkness gives way to light as we step forth with strength and joy. We have returned, like the prodigal son, from the far country. It is a new day. It is a new life. It is a time to be healed.

In His Image and Likeness

What is the chief object of man? To glorify God in his body; this is the true answer. Have the courage to make the heroic attempt to give personal expression to God. Charles Fillmore's words are aflame with ardor and conviction. It *does* take courage to pursue life uncompromisingly so that the glory of God can have unlimited expression in our bodies and souls. Perhaps the real heroes of this world, when all is said and done, will be those who dare to take their stands with the Almighty. *" . . . not my will, but thine, be done,"* (Luke 22:42) *thy* will in my soul and body.

And what is the will of God? It is always perfection and good. It cannot be otherwise, for God is only good, a Creator whose very nature it is to persistently and continuously seek self-expression in the physical world. And so He created us. In us He placed His hopes for perfection and permanence, bestowing upon us the divine potential for achieving that perfection and permanence.

This universal life force within us has an insatiable desire for wholeness. It dwells in every cell of our bodies and seeks to manifest and express life. This is God at work within the very membranes of our cells, whispering in our ears, urging us toward perfection.

Life Force Is Universal

This mysterious life force in our bodies is the same universal force that holds the planets in their orbits, causes the tides to rise and fall, brings forth the sequoia from the tiny seed, and propels an amoeba through a drop of water. And the direction of this force, this Spirit, is always toward the good, an eternal quest for perfection and the awareness of the complete unity of all life.

That there is such a Spirit omnipresent is evidenced on every hand in the so-called healing power of nature. It is constantly healing and restoring the cut, bruised, and broken in all creation.

The mark of the woodsman's ax on the forest tree is as carefully healed as is the cut on the finger of the little child. The healing Spirit is no respecter of persons or things, but does its work effectively wherever and whenever it has the opportunity. (Charles Fillmore)

Spiritual and Scientific Synthesis

Metaphysicians find it easy and natural to believe in the healing life force. What is remarkable today, however, is the prodigious corroboration of these beliefs coming from the world of science! Everywhere around us we see evidence of the synthesis of the spiritual and the scientific. It is all coming together, and why shouldn't it? Are we not all searching for the same answer? Are not science and religion both addressing themselves, ultimately, to the same questions: Who are we? From where did we come?

Here are the words of Doctor Albert Szent-Györgyi, one of the world's greatest biochemists, a two-time recipient of the Nobel Prize, who admits that he has spent his life *in the hunt for the secret of life.* He, too, sees the life force as an intelligent Spirit seeking wholeness. *My feeling is that living matter carries, in itself, a hitherto undefined principle, a tendency for perfecting itself.* These lines were written in 1963. Later, this same highly respected scientist began to use the word *drive* instead of *tendency.* And today we find

317

him saying things like this: *Since I was not afraid to use the word "drive," I might as well be even more audacious and use the word "wisdom." I am not the first to do so.* He adds that it is *a really remarkable wisdom* and one which might be the very factor that *has driven matter to generate life.* Doctor Szent-Györgyi concludes with a moving revelation of his own awe of the life force, resulting from half a century of research and probing, which endowed him with *such a speechless deep reverence and amazement before the wonders of nature.*

Isn't it obvious that we are all going in the same direction, religionists and scientists alike? There is little doubt in the minds of either that everything in the universe operates according to law, a law greater than ourselves, and yet a law of which each of us is a part. And we, when we work *with* the law, can do indescribably wondrous things. We can do the *"even greater works"* of which Jesus Christ spoke. We can limitlessly unfold our potential, letting our true God nature express fully in our souls and bodies.

Working with the Law

The secret of perfection is working *with* the law. Law may manifest as spiritual laws and physical laws, as we all realize, but they are all part of the one law. They are all part of God. The universe is one. Therefore, disobeying physical laws carries the same judgment as disobeying spiritual laws. We might not consider stealing from our neighbor or telling a lie, for instance, and yet we may not hesitate to poison the life force within our cells by eating harmful foods. Stealing, lying, and eating harmful foods are sins against the law. The fact that one is spiritual and one is physical does not matter. How could it if *everything* is God? And since everything works according to the law of God, it is subject to the same judgment. The "crime" always carries with it its own punishment. Disobeying a spiritual law brings damage and disorder to the soul. Disobeying a physical law brings damage and disorder to the body.

The same compassion that we so freely give to the lives of others must also be freely given to the life in our own bodies. *Have compassion on the life in the body of every living creature, and especially in your own body,* said Charles Fillmore. We must not hurt life, ours or another's, because life is God.

Triune Man

Perhaps this book has brought you to a new path. Perhaps some spark of illumination regarding humanity's divine potential has been kindled.

We have seen how we must nourish equally the triune aspects of man—Spirit, soul, and body. And we have seen not only the necessity of this nourishment but also some of the various means of providing it.

We have seen that the life force can be approached in several ways. If there is a healing need, we deal with it spiritually first because we know that our health is the result of how much of our true Christ self we are able to recognize and manifest. (We do not deny the appearance of a condition but, rather, we deny any power in that condition. Certainly the condition seems to exist, else why would we be trying to overcome it?)

We must realize, however, that all conditions, no matter how undesirable they may appear, are expressions of God. They are *limited* expressions, to be sure, but expressions nonetheless. We can improve these expressions through prayer and meditation, proper nutrition, physical exercise, and even medication if we feel it necessary. (Medical science assists nature by diminishing the power of the disease, thereby giving the healing life force the opportunity to come forward and do its mighty work.)

Holistic Health

Myrtle Fillmore (like Charles) was ahead of her time with her holistic view of health. *Healing will come through taking the right mental attitude, and getting right down into the body and telling it the Truth; then following up this treatment daily with really sensible and scientific living habits. Supply the foods that are needed, so that the bloodstream can be clean and vital and enabled to do its work of washing out the accumulations and rebuilding and perfecting the muscles, and nerves, and bones, and tissues.*

We have learned that the proper foods to supply the body temple are the top-grade proteins, the constructive carbohydrates, and good oils. Each meal, including breakfast, should contain these.

In addition, we have seen the benefits to be derived from supplemental vitamins and minerals.

We have learned that junk foods (sugar, white flour, and all of the nefarious "goodies" made from them), alcohol, tobacco, and narcotics do not belong in the body. Like the money changers and merchants of Jerusalem, they should be cast out of the temple, for the "temple" is the sacred dwelling place of God.

"But don't take away my goodies!" some will exclaim. "They taste so good." Yes, they do. But should that really matter? We have to come to realize that when we take away our "goodies" (which would be more aptly named "baddies!") we begin to take away arthritis, diabetes, high blood pressure, and all of the other ills that plague humankind.

Richard Lynch in his inspiring book, *The Secret of*

Health, says: *There is no greater or more important work for you in the universe than the discovery of your real self.* When we can grasp the motivating power of these words, we begin to take seriously the physical laws that God designed for preserving the body temple. Food no longer is a social happening, served to impress others with its sensations of taste or visual effects. It becomes instead a sacrament, a sanctified ritual to the glory of the divine life force which never slackens in its fervent dedication to keeping us alive. We recognize food as the hallowed nourishment that the life force utilizes to create the perfect flesh of our bodies. And so we do our best to provide the highest quality nourishment possible, knowing that the structure can only be as good as the raw materials that went into it.

Body Prosperity

True body prosperity is what we seek. A beautiful soul deserves an equally beautiful body in which to reside, not a hovel, but a palace befitting the royalty of the divine creation known as man. Good nutrition contributes to body prosperity, and so does physical exercise.

One of the major differences between the living and the nonliving is the ability of the living to improve itself. The nonliving (automobiles, clothes, furniture, etc.) is worn out by use. The living is improved and developed by use. To remain alive life must keep going, building up and improving itself. Inactivity, nonuse, makes it fail and fall apart.

The necessity for regular body exercise is one of the basic physical laws. That which is constantly improved cannot perish!

Courage and Heroism

Spirit, soul, and body—the totality of man, the magnificent. How *fearfully and wonderfully* are we made! How perfectly in every way the great Creator fashioned us out of Himself. What unspeakable love must have gone into our creation. What undreamed of hopes of the Almighty must lie deep within our beings. What expectations of unlimited greatness must be heaped upon us.

Let us rise up and serve the Lord in the only way we can, by perfecting our bodies and souls until they are eternally one with Spirit. Let us *have the courage to make the heroic attempt* of which Charles Fillmore spoke.

The time is past when we can expect God to change us. God has already done for us all He can do. He has given us everything. If we want to evolve into something higher, then it is we who will have to make the effort. Our future is in *our* hands.

When we work with the law, we have the power to achieve anything and everything, including unlimited physical perfection. The choice is ours: Adam, or Christ, or anything in between. The life force will not fail us. Let us totally nourish it so we can begin to discover our true destinies and manifest that divine design in which we were created—the image and likeness of God!

Printed U.S.A.
162-F-7697-10M-4-85